Creative Approaches in Dementia Care

Edited by

Hilary Lee
and
Trevor Adams

palgrave
macmillan

Contents

List of table and figures

Table

Figures

Foreword

'There is no use trying,' said Alice. 'One can't believe impossible things.' 'I daresay you haven't had much practice,' said the Queen. 'When I was your age, I always did it for half an hour a day. Why, sometimes I've believed as many as six impossible things before breakfast.'
— Lewis Carroll, Through the Looking Glass

What is creativity? Photographer Dewitt Jones (1999) defines it as 'a moment – a moment where we look at the ordinary, but see the extraordinary'. This simple definition describes what is so important about this book.

Our traditional view of dementia is one that focuses on loss – loss of nerve cells, memory and impairments in various types of cognition. We constantly measure people living with dementia by what they cannot do. Standardized assessments like the Folstein Mini-Mental Status Exam are a litany of discrete tasks to be performed: Can you spell 'world' backwards? Can you remember three objects after five minutes? Can you copy a figure of two intersecting pentagons?

In performing these assessments, we reduce the person to the sum of those discrete tasks. This distracts us from the fact that many complex and integrative skills continue to exist, even in advanced forms of the illness. Our focus on disease and deficits blinds us to seeing the whole person. This biased view – referred to by Kitwood (1997) as 'positioning' – leads us to respond to expressions of distress or need by blaming neuropathology, rather than looking into the heart of the person in our care.

In our biomedical approach to dementia, we have created care environments around the needs of well care-partners, rather than those of the person living with dementia. In explaining the fallacy of this approach, I often ask audiences to think of a man whose legs have become paralysed, who now needs a wheelchair for mobility. Through tireless advocacy,

new laws have been enacted requiring building owners to con-
struct ramps and other types of disability access, in order to
enable such a person to continue to succeed in our world.

But we don't build 'ramps' for people with dementia. We
create environments where they can no longer succeed, and
blame the resultant distress on their 'disease'. Imagine push-
ing the man I just described out of his wheelchair and exhort-
ing him to 'walk as we do'. Next, imagine that after he falls to
the ground and becomes angry with us, we diagnose a 'behaviour problem' and give him a sedating medication. It sounds
ludicrous, but we do this every day to people who live with
dementia, in all care environments around the world.

In crafting a new 'experiential' view of dementia that
enables engagement and growth, I use a simple definition:
Dementia is 'a shift in the person's perception of the world'
(Power, 2010). By moving our focus from disease to shifting
experience, it is possible to see the whole person and conceive
of new approaches to care that reflect and capitalize upon how
that individual sees the world.

Once we have re-framed our view of dementia and shifted
our focus from *disability* to *possibility*, it is easier to see the
intersection of creativity with dementia. In fact, Jones's definition of creativity seems to embrace the very core experience
of the person living with dementia: looking at the ordinary,
but seeing the extraordinary. Instead of simply viewing such a
shift as evidence of confused pathology, is it possible to channel this perspective through creative expression and enhance
one's well-being as a result? This book answers that question
with a resounding 'Yes!'

The first lesson for creativity is that it is a trait we all possess.
The ability to see the world around us with 'new eyes' exists
in every person, each according to his or her perspective. This
ability does not end with a diagnosis of dementia; in fact, the
mind's detachment from ordinary patterns of thinking may
actually enhance one's ability to untether the creative spirit.

And that is also what creativity is – a *spirit* that is ignited
when the mind is fully engaged in the genesis of new thoughts.
There is an inherent joy in beholding something that you have
conceived in your own way. That is why a songwriter can perform the same repertoire night after night without becoming

bored. Each performance is a rediscovery of the creative process, magnified by the energy felt when those around you share your creation.

Another lesson is that creativity transcends language. The loss of speech that can occur with dementia is not a barrier to ongoing creativity. On the contrary, disrupted patterns of speech can create new words, 'neologisms' that express multiple meanings and emotions in novel ways. *'Twas brillig and the slithy toves did gyre and gimble in the wabe'.* When Carroll wrote this, we called it genius; when people with dementia speak this way, we call it nonsense.

Furthermore, engaging the creative arts can activate pathways that release thoughts and words previously held captive by broken circuitry. There are millions of 'back doors' to communication that can be opened with a non-traditional approach, be it art, music, visual stimulus, tactile sensation, humour or strong emotion. This book abounds with stories of such successes.

Many of us are hampered by our own paradigms – it is the individual who can break free of these established patterns of thought and find new discoveries. In his 1942 novel *Pilote de Guerre,* Antoine de St. Exupery wrote, 'A rock pile ceases to be a rock pile the moment a single man contemplates it, bearing within him the image of a cathedral.' When the mind is freed of mundane thought patterns, there are new worlds to discover. We can learn much about imagination from people who live with dementia.

Perhaps the most important lesson of creativity is that it exists *in the moment.* A learned scholar or accomplished artist may read past writings, work through complex formulae or practice her art, but when the creative spark hits, it triggers a process that unfolds in the mindfulness of present.

Once again, dementia can provide the perfect palette for painting the creative landscape. Unfettered from the weight of memory, people living with dementia exist more and more in the present moment. As memory dims and reminiscence becomes less durable, engagement in the moment is often the best approach to creating well-being.

In the creative moment, there are no rules and regulations. There is no 'right answer'. There is not even a need to *be* right, because every next moment promises another opportunity for renewal. People living with dementia also teach us about mindfulness.

One last lesson about creativity is that it contradicts the common wisdom about 'limited brain reserve'. Just as the letters of the alphabet can be displayed in infinite variety, so can our range of creative expression. In this way, the creative process is like a muscle – it becomes more powerful and versatile with repeated use.

Recent research has brought to question our long-held medical beliefs that 'nerve cells don't regenerate' and 'brain damage is permanent'. Kitwood (1997) coined the term 'rementing' for his theory that a nourishing care environment can create new brain growth and capabilities, even in the face of advanced dementia. This concept was met with a great deal of skepticism then; it doesn't seem so impossible now.

Indeed, people living with dementia are learning every day, incorporating names, places and many of the positive and negative experiences of their daily life and care. We tend not to see this because we focus on deficits, but *what if our focus shifted to cultivating strengths through creative engagement?* What often results is nothing less than a virtual 'reversal' of many of those deficits associated with dementia. Here's why: There are two disabilities of dementia. The first is a result of damage to brain cells, which at present remains irreversible. But there is another hidden disability: the *excess disability* caused by a care approach that positions, disempowers, isolates and overmedicates the person. Creative engagement enables us to remove much of this excess disability, and people come to life with new abilities thought to be long lost to their illness. The following chapters on the *Spark of Life* approach and a multitude of other creative endeavours will demonstrate the frequency and durability of these 'awakenings'.

In a 2005 monograph, Fox et al. described seven domains of well-being: *identity, growth, autonomy, security, connectedness, meaning and joy.* In addition to being universal across ages and cultures, these domains can also exist independent of one's cognitive or functional abilities, *if* they are recognized and cultivated by the care environment.

As you read the following chapters, it will become strikingly apparent that well-facilitated engagement through the creative arts can feed all seven domains of well-being simultaneously, reigniting one's spirit even in the latter stages of dementia. If I could create a pill that did this, I would likely be a Nobel laureate and a very rich man. But I will wager that such a pill will never exist, as neither creativity nor well-being can be bottled.

Before you turn the page, I will offer one last quote (from Sheik Ahmed Zaki Yamani) about creativity and possibility, to enhance your journey:

'The Stone Age didn't end because they ran out of stones.'

G. ALLEN POWER, MD, FACP
Rochester, NY, USA
15 August 2010

References

Carroll, L. (1926). *Through the Looking Glass* (originally published in 1865). New York: Macmillan.

Fox, N., Norton, L., Rashap, A. W. et al. (2005). Well-being: beyond quality of life (unpublished monograph, obtainable from info@ edenalt.org).

Jones, D. (1999). *Everyday Creativity* (motion picture). (Available from Star Thrower Distribution, 26 East Exchange St., Suite 600, St. Paul, MN 55101).

Kitwood, T. (1997). *Dementia Reconsidered: The Person Comes First.* New York: Open University Press.

Power, G. A. (2010). *Dementia beyond Drugs: Changing the Culture of Care.* Baltimore: Health Professions Press.

St. Exupéry, A. d. (1942). *Pilote de Guerre.* Paris: Gallimard.

Yamani, A. Z. (21 August 2005). Quoted in *The Breaking Point*, by Peter Maass. *The New York Times Magazine.*

Acknowledgements

I would like to express my appreciation to the chapter authors for the heart and soul they have put into the creation of this book. Special thanks go to all the people with dementia whose stories, life journeys and wisdom are shared to give us all profound insights. I would like to extend my gratitude to the team at Palgrave Macmillan for their guidance and support through the compilation of this book. Finally, my deep appreciation goes to my family for their understanding, love and patience through the many hours spent in the process of writing and editing.

Hilary Lee

Dedicated to Thomas and Jonathan Adams, my sons who always encourage and inspire me.

Trevor Adams

The editors and publisher also wish to thank the following for permission to use copyright material

Notes on contributors

Trevor Adams is a Lecturer and Strategic Lead, Dementia Care, Division of Health and Social Care, University of Surrey, UK. He is qualified in general, mental health and community mental health nursing and has worked in dementia care for over 30 years. He specializes in dementia care nursing and has written numerous papers, chapters in academic journals and books, including co-editing four books on dementia care. Trevor has gained a national and international reputation in his field, having spoken at over 50 conferences in the United Kingdom, Europe, Canada and Australia. He is an Associate Editor of *Dementia: The International Journal of Social Research and Practice* and holds honorary fellowships with the University of Brighton and Christ Church University, Canterbury, UK.

Kate Allan's background is in clinical psychology, and her interest in the subject of communication and creativity with persons with dementia has involved undertaking work in the areas of service-user consultation, the combination of deafness and communication with persons with very advanced dementia. She is particularly interested in exploring how creative activities can help both people with dementia and their supporters to flourish and is herself a keen practitioner of various fibre arts. She is now a freelance consultant and trainer in the field of dementia and has written and spoken widely about her work. She continues to practise as a clinical psychologist.

Patricia Baines brings to her art therapy praxis both the closeness of the participant observer and the insights of the clinician, bringing together training as a psychologist with many years of working as an anthropologist. For the past eight years she has been working with individuals living with dementia for Alzheimer's Australia Tasmania. She has made many presentations at international and national conferences on the value of employing art therapy with individuals with many different diseases, which cause dementia. Her own painting and writing provide a source of ongoing inspiration and replenishment for her therapeutic work.

Richard Coaten is a Dance Movement Psychotherapist with the South West Yorkshire Partnership NHS Foundation Trust and runs a Dance Movement Psychotherapy Service in Calderdale. An experienced arts therapist and dancer, his special interests are in older people with memory problems. Richard has a doctoral thesis from Roehampton University, is familiar with current research, practice and literature and the need to support the development and training of dancers who work in this field. He has published work and has delivered significant arts-based training programs over the years. He receives a Winston Churchill Travelling Fellowship (2010) to study embodied practices in Canada.

Joanna Jaaniste is a registered Dramatherapist who has practised in mental health and substance abuse for 16 years. More recently, she enjoys working with elderly people and especially with individuals who have dementia. Joanna believes strongly in dramatherapy's power to assist participants to find new meaning in their lives, and to assist elders with existential questions. She is the principal of the Dramatherapy Centre in Sydney, has taught at postgraduate level and is now studying for a PhD. She has presented papers in UK, USA and South Africa and has published articles in a variety of journals.

Kirsten James is a registered nurse and qualified educator who has been nursing for almost 30 years and working in dementia care for the past 10 years. She has qualifications and has worked with Complementary Therapies in aged, dementia and palliative care, and this has led to her contributing to nursing curricula, textbooks, journals and research in the field. She has also presented at numerous seminars, conferences and workshops in both the community and tertiary sectors. In 2006, she was awarded a state government Nursing Excellence Award that recognized that Complementary Therapies improved the quality of life of the residents that she and her team cared for. She is currently working as a consultant with the Dementia Behaviour Management Advisory Service Victoria, Australia.

John Killick was a teacher of English and drama for 30 years but has been a writer all his life. He worked in a women's prison and a hospice before becoming Writer in Residence for Westminster Health Care. Here he first encountered people with dementia, and began to produce poems from their words. He has now published three books of poetry. Since then he has undertaken work exploring many creative activities with persons with dementia and is currently involved in improvisatory drama work with people in Scotland. He has lectured, broadcast and written widely on these subjects both in the UK and abroad.

Trisha Kotai-Ewers has a BA in languages and an MPhil in Medieval and Renaissance Studies from the University of Western Australia. For 25 years she taught languages in government and independent schools in Western Australian. She is completing a PhD on the history of the Fellowship of Australian Writers, WA, with which she has been involved since 1988. In 1997, Trisha began working as Writer in Residence with people with dementia and has given papers on her work at national and international conferences. In 2007, the Alzheimer's Association, WA, published her book *Listen to the Talk of Us: People with dementia speak out.*

Hilary Lee is President and Co-Founder of *Spark of Life* World Foundation, with a global focus on education, research and innovation. She has a background in occupational therapy and has completed a Master's in Science at Curtin University of Technology in Perth, Australia, researching the outcomes of the *Spark of Life* Club Program. Hilary has undertaken many projects in dementia care that have been the first of their kind and has presented her work both nationally and internationally. These include easing the transition to residential care, the early identification and prevention of depression in people with dementia and a multidisciplinary approach to palliative care. Hilary recently completed a study on creative expression in dementia developing a new assessment tool in collaboration with researchers at the University of British Columbia. Hilary founded the Society for the Arts in Dementia Care (Australia) Inc. in 2006, a chapter of the Canadian society originally established by Dr Dalia Gottlieb-Tanaka.

Elizabeth MacKinlay is a registered nurse and priest in the Anglican Church and Director of the Centre for Ageing and Pastoral Studies, St Mark's National Theological Centre, Canberra, and Professor in the School of Theology, Charles Sturt University. An active researcher and writer, Elizabeth has presented many papers and workshops, both nationally and internationally. Elizabeth is editor of the new book *Ageing and Spirituality across Faiths and Cultures*, 2010, following soon after the release of the Japanese version of *Facilitating Spiritual Reminiscence in People with Dementia*.

Kirstin Robertson-Gillam is a Music Therapist, registered nurse, counsellor and educator with experience in aged and palliative care, mental health and disabilities. She gives mentor supervision to students, graduate music therapists and coun-sellors. She created Spirited Living Meditations® which utilizes imagery, music and meditation for people of all ages to moti-vate and improve health. Kirstin holds a BA in Psychology and Musicology, a Master's in Counselling and MA(Hons) in research. She is a PhD candidate (UWS), researching the con-nection between singing to alleviate depression in older popu-lations. She does sessional EAP and WorkCover counselling as well as delivering education in aged care and music therapy.

Pam Schweitzer has spent the past 30 years developing remi-niscence work in the UK and across Europe. She founded Age Exchange Theatre Trust in 1983 and was its Artistic Director for 23 years. She created the first Reminiscence Centre in London in 1987 and in 1993, she established the European Reminiscence Network. For the Network, she has coordinated international festivals and conferences and initiated collabora-tive action research projects. 'Remembering Yesterday, Caring Today', a reminiscence project for people with dementia and their family carers, was piloted across Europe in 1997 and has since been continuously developed and refined. Pam Schweitzer is currently a consultant and freelance practitioner in the fields of arts and older people, communication in dementia care, intercultural work and international cooperation on creative projects. She is an Honorary Research Fellow at Greenwich University.

Peter Spitzer is the Principal in a General Practice in Bowral, New South Wales, Australia. He is the Founding Chairman, Medical Director and a co-Founder of the Humour Foundation charity. The Humour Foundation Clown Doctor program is national, and he regularly visits paediatric as well as general hospitals and palliative care facilities. He lectures and presents workshops on 'Humour in Practice' to health care professionals. His work has also been presented overseas. Articles have been published in medical journals and the media. In 2003 he developed the LaughterBoss concept in aged care and presented this at 'The 1st National Conference on Challenging Depression in Aged Care' in Sydney, Australia. He is involved in a landmark, 3-year (2009–2011), NH&MRC-funded SMILE Study to research the impact of humour therapy in dementia care. He delights in being an Australia Day Ambassador.

Jane Verity is the Founder of Dementia Care Australia and *Spark of Life*, and a world leader and pioneer in the emotional care of people with dementia. She has the vision and courage to challenge the status quo and create a world of dementia care that ignites the human spirit. Jane is also Co-Founder of the *Spark of Life* World Foundation. Originally from Denmark and now living in Australia, Jane is an Occupational and Family Therapist, a Master Practitioner in Neuro Linguistic Programming (NLP) and has earned the highest international accreditation as a professional speaker. Jane is known for her life-changing and inspirational presentations and has reached audiences all around the world. She has authored two internationally published books and contributes regularly to national and international dementia conferences and journals.

Introduction

Hilary Lee and Trevor Adams

Dr Richard Taylor, who has Alzheimer's disease, in addressing the conference of Alzheimer's Disease International in Singapore, 2009, called on the dementia care leaders in the audience to put psychosocial interventions onto the priority list so that people living with dementia might have their emotional needs understood and met, 'We are millions living with dementia right now and we need your help to lead meaningful and fulfilling lives, while we are waiting for a cure' (Power et al., 2009).

The topic of this book responds to this heartfelt plea so powerfully expressed by Richard Taylor. The topic also fits within the new paradigm of placing the person first that is currently evolving in the health and care of people with dementia. This underlying approach of person-centred care combined with new insights from the frontiers of creative arts and science to enhance the health of mind, body and spirit combined. Recent research shows us that as the brain remains plastic, new or compensatory learning can still occur in dementia, so when we use creativity we can not only support improvement in abilities but also create a life worth living for people with dementia (Power, 2010).

Person-centred dementia care

The development of person-centred care in the 1990s began a change from a medically orientated focus on the disease to a supportive and individualized approach focusing on the whole person. This approach provides a strong theoretical foundation for the use of creative arts in dementia care. Person-centred care was initially developed by Professor Tom Kitwood, Founder 'of the Bradford Dementia Group, University of Bradford, United Kingdom. Kitwood was a visionary advocate for people with dementia and those involved in their care, and his work has underpinned progressive thinking on dementia care for the past 20 years. He challenged the idea that the bio-medical model of illness was the only way of viewing people with dementia (Kitwood, 1997). Kitwood believed that seeing people with dementia in medical terms led them to be seen as objects with neither identity nor personhood. He pointed out that people's experience of dementia arises not only from their degree of neurological impairment and their physical health but also from social and psychological factors including their personal biography and day-to-day interaction with other people.

Person-centred care addresses the impact of social environment and quality of our interaction with the person who has dementia rather than the disease process itself. Person-centred creative approaches highlight the need for individualized support for the person with dementia. In addition, as this book demonstrates, it is the quality of our interaction, and our way of thinking and being while we facilitate creative expression that forms the key to unlocking the potential of people with dementia.

Kitwood (1997) described the task of good dementia care as

* sustaining personhood of each individual in the face of advancing cognitive impairment;
* understanding that people with dementia rely on everyone in their surroundings to guarantee, replenish and uphold their personhood.

Personhood is different from personality and Kitwood described it as a person

* having valid experience;
* living in relationships and
* being an originating source of activity. (Kitwood, 1998)

He defined it further as 'a standing or a status that is bestowed on one human being, by another in the context of relationship and social being' (Kitwood, 1997, p. 8). Kitwood also took a moral position, seeing personhood as sacred and unique. He shifted the focus from viewing people with dementia purely in terms of the disease to seeing them as sentient beings with an ethical and valued status thus emphasizing our obligation 'to treat each other with deep respect' (ibid.). Within person-centred care it is acknowledged that the personal and social identity of a person with dementia arises in and is supported by their social environment (including the arts).

For Kitwood, personhood becomes apparent when communication takes place, and he outlined 17 different interactive processes that may occur in dementia care settings which undermine personhood. He called these the malignant social psychology. His choice of the word 'malignant' emphasizes the harmful impact of these behaviours on the person with dementia. One type of malignant social psychology is 'outpacing' which occurs when information is provided at a rate that is too fast for a person to process or understand. Another is 'disruption' or breaking a person's frame of reference. This occurs when there is a sudden intrusion or disruption to a person's action. For example, a person may be engaged in a creative process, such as painting, when a staff member suddenly interrupts to carry out a routine task, taking them out of the room and thereby stopping their creative flow and thoughts.

Kitwood (1997) observed ten different types of good communication that promote personhood, which he calls 'positive person work'. One form of positive person work is 'timalation' which occurs when the person with dementia encounters sensory experiences such as those that are offered by the creative arts. Another form of positive person work is 'play'. Play is central to all creativity, in fact without play there is no creativity (Estes, 1992). According to Kitwood (1993), two more positive person work concepts, 'holding' and 'facilitation' enable a higher level of communication between carer and the person with dementia, enabling cooperation and a reciprocal engagement. He explained that with successful communication the person with dementia feels recognized as a person, self-esteem is enhanced, social confidence increases and hope is sustained. Rather than making extra demands on the caregiver, this approach can transform care-causing exhaustion to providing stimulation and refreshment.

Five core psychological needs of people with dementia were identified by Kitwood (1997). He depicted these as five petals of a flower with love as the centre. The petals represent inclusion, attachment, comfort, identity and occupation. It is essential that all these psychological needs are sustained by everyone who is supporting a person with dementia. Creative arts' facilitators play a vital role in meeting these core psychological needs. When warmth and love is part of their attitude, they will profoundly support the emotional well-being of their clients with dementia. The chapters of this book provide many examples of how the core psychological needs can be met in different ways when the person with dementia takes part in creative arts programs and projects. For example, singing in a choir may provide a person with all of the core psychological needs. Inclusion (and therefore belonging) comes from being part of a close group that meets for a common purpose. Attachment develops as the choir members form friendships and become close as a result of their regular meetings and common interest. Comfort is facilitated in a safe psychological environment through the loving, empowering and caring approach of the choir leader. The identity of choir members develops through their relationships with both the other members and the community where they sing because of the recognition that they gain. In addition, identity is supported by the common purpose, with the knowledge that each person makes a valid and valuable contribution towards the success of the whole choir. Finally, group singing provides meaningful occupation where members can creatively express deep feelings.

The intention of this book is to give health care practitioners and students and anyone who cares for people with dementia a unique reference to a range of creative approaches that will open up new opportunities for dementia care. The focus is not on the diagnosis or types of dementia, instead the book explores practical, and innovative creative psychosocial approaches. Although the book does not claim to enable readers to practise these approaches, as each one represents an area of speciality that may take years to learn, there may be elements or ideas that practitioners can be inspired to use in their everyday care of people with dementia. International experts and pioneers in their own fields, provide an overview of their work, highlighting its value, and evidence-based theoretical frameworks, with some practical suggestions as to how they can be accessed and implemented.

This book provides a unique collection of a wide and diverse variety of creative approaches and the arts which go outside the boundaries of conventional thinking about dementia care. These include the *Spark of Life* Concept, the LaughterBoss (therapeutic use of humour), art, dramatherapy, storytelling, dance movement psychotherapy, photography, creative reminiscence work, videography, complementary therapies, spirituality and creative communication in the late stage of dementia.

Creativity

Dr Dalia Gottlieb-Tanaka has explored the nature of creativity for people with dementia in her doctoral research. She defines creativity as follows:

> Creativity in the context of dementia adds something new and different to the world whether through intrinsic self-exploration as an individual, or sharing creative expression through interaction with others. The creative process is demonstrated through creative thinking and imagination in everyday living and may or may not result in a product. Through creativity, people with dementia could (can) enjoy meaningful, satisfying and (at times) unpredictable experiences that may last for only a very short while or as long as memory allows it. (Gottlieb-Tanaka, 2006, p. 43)

Creativity and personhood

Creativity has a strong value within person-centred care because it enables the strengthening and expression of personhood while also providing opportunities for enriched relationships. According to Kasayka (2002, p. 9), the core functions of the expressive arts are 'the reclamation, the regeneration and the celebration of the human spirit', the same primary goals of person-centred care. This quote comes from *Healing Arts Therapies in Person-Centred Care* which pioneered new insights into how the arts (music, dance and art, in this book) could form part of Kitwood's positive person work. Celebration of the human spirit is a theme that is brought to life in many of the chapters of this book, as the authors demonstrate the power of creative approaches to bring out each person's unique spirituality and the expression of their spirit or essence.

A decade ago the culture of care and the medical world paid little attention to how people with dementia viewed their condition (Kotai-Ewers, 2007), but more recently through the development of person-centred care and an expansion of interest in the creative arts, health professionals now have begun to truly hear and appreciate the point of view of people with dementia. The creative process enables people with dementia to affirm their identity and validate their thoughts and feelings by expressing what is deeply meaningful to them. Through creativity they can share with others wisdom and stories they have gained throughout their lives. These expressions often take health professionals, family members and carers by surprise and provide deep insights into what the person with dementia is really experiencing. Creative communication with love and empathy can be extremely powerful and awaken dormant abilities that have been suppressed through traditional biomedical approaches towards dementia (Power et al., 2009).

Creativity connects people

Natalie Rogers (1993) points out how something magical happens when people work side by side, and how through companionship ideas and creativity are stimulated.

By offering new ways of expression to people with dementia, the creative arts give life and provide a powerful link between their inner and outer world. Rogers describes creativity as a bridge to the inner self, connecting us to our bodies, our senses and facilitating a journey in self-discovery and personal growth. She describes how by channelling emotions into expressive arts, people can gain a deeper appreciation of their worth and release negative emotions. Creativity can also bring generations together, helping them gain deep insights about each other and forge new connections with people that make life both meaningful and joyful (Lee, 2005, 2006). Creating human connection through the creative arts also has a positive value in preventing or reducing depression in dementia care. This can be achieved through the positive relationships and friendships developed during the sharing of a project with others or through the opportunities to express personal thoughts, feelings and stories in a safe psychological environment (Lee, 2007; Lee & Blades, 2007). Creativity gives hope to those diagnosed with dementia because it not only offers opportunities to provide meaningful communication but also enables health care professionals to focus on a person's strengths rather than their limitations (Abraham, 2005).

Creativity enables improvement

According to Gottlieb-Tanaka (2006) person-centred care enables us to look at creativity as providing opportunities instead of focusing on the disabilities of people with dementia. She shows that creativity can enhance cognition, physical abilities, behaviour and enable new social responses to an enriched creative environment. Oliver Sachs in his book *Musicophelia* explains that music has healing benefits for cognition, and identity, even for those with advanced dementia because 'musical perception, musical sensitivity, musical emotion and musical memory can survive long after other forms of memory have disappeared' (Sachs, 2007, p. 337).

Swiss art therapist Beat Ted Hannermann (2006) argues that people with dementia are capable of improving their creative skills, sharpening their senses and strengthening their propensity to act themselves. Older people are often able to develop their ability of improvisation and imagination to a higher degree than younger people because of their more extensive experiences in life (Hannermann, 2006). Neurogenesis is still possible in old age according to psychiatrist and researcher Norman Doidge (2007). Doidge explains that even when the brain of an older person is going through a significant deterioration, it can still undergo a vast plastic reorganization which could help compensate for the brain's losses. Creativity reinforces essential connections between brain cells, including those that activate memory (Cohen, 2000). Through creativity people with dementia can regain dormant abilities thought lost, such as communication skills, the ability to remember stories and other events, desire for social contact and interest in life (Lee, 2007). The therapeutic effects of laughter (for example, the work of the LaughterBoss as described in Chapter 3) have been shown to have lasting mental and physical benefits as demonstrated in psychoneuroimmunology studies (Spitzer, 2008).

Conditions that foster creativity

Natalie Rogers, the daughter of Carl Rogers (the humanist who formulated the foundations of person-centred care), described the external conditions that foster and nurture the internal conditions for creativity. The first two are from Carl Rogers and the third is from Natalie:

1. Psychological safety
   a) Accepting the individual as of unconditional worth;
   b) Providing a climate in which external evaluation is absent;
   c) Understanding empathetically.
2. Psychological freedom
3. Offering stimulating and challenging experiences (Rogers, 1993, p. 14).

Having a safe, non-judgemental psychological space for creative expression is vital to free feelings and ideas. Accepting the individual as having unconditional worth is achieved when the facilitator conveys their belief 'that each individual is precious regardless of any present words or behaviour' (Rogers, 1993, p. 15). Providing an environment where external evaluation is absent contributes to providing a safe psychological space, freeing the person to be who they are and knowing there are no winners or losers, and each person's contribution is genuinely valued. Inspired by her father, Natalie Rogers highlights the importance of providing psychological freedom for symbolic expression of feelings and ideas through the creative arts. Finally, Rogers shares her insight that creative experiences need to be carefully planned by the facilitator to offer stimulating and challenging experiences. This notion is supported by the work of Mihaly Csikszentmihalyi, the Hungarian psychologist who created the theory of flow. Flow is the process for achieving happiness through control over one's inner life and how life can still be enjoyed despite adversity. Csikszentmihalyi (1992) found that as humans we need a balance between healthy challenges that stretch us and enable us to grow and the skills we have to meet those challenges.

Overview of the chapters

The *Spark of Life* Concept outlined in Chapter 1 offers both a powerful approach and framework for creative expression that builds on person-centred foundations as well as occupational science and neurolinguistic programming. The Concept is both philosophical and practical, and it also facilitates the finding of meaning in life at a profoundly deep level with a focus on the well-being of the human spirit. The positive and meaningful experiences in the safe psychological environment promoted through the concept contribute to a feeling of belonging, closeness and friendship that has a healing effect for people with dementia. In addition, the concept can be applied using creative learning processes with the entire care team, working towards enriching the organizational culture and environment.

The approach of blending art and science with love and compassion to lift the spirits of people with dementia is further explored in Peter Spitzer's chapter (Chapter 2). He describes the LaughterBoss concept as a modern day court jester which facilitates therapeutic humour in aged care facilities. Spitzer gives us the evidence for humour being good for our health – for our mind, body and spirit – with some practical examples of good practice. The value of humour is scientifically supported with supporting research as well as true case studies and practical examples.

Dramatherapy and dementia care by Joanna Jaaniste (Chapter 3) provides some deep insights into the value of dramatherapy in dementia care, which is as yet an underutilized expressive art form. She gives practitioners some very practical ideas to achieve success using drama with people with dementia. Jaaniste has illuminated on how to use dramatherapy with puppets, play, storytelling and improvisation. This author also highlights the importance of psychological safety and trust, ensuring that participants have the opportunity for reflection at the end of the session to share any uncomfortable feelings or memories that may have been stirred.

Personhood can be embodied, and this concept is explored in great depth in Richard Coaten's dance movement therapy chapter (Chapter 4). He explores and develops the significance of embodied practices as being of value in developing relationships, improving mobility, affirming identity and supporting effective communication. Coaten also illustrates how movement and dance contribute embodied pathways that provide a powerful link between the person and their experience of the world.

Creativity provides a new language that is liberated from the need to find words. Kirstin Robertson-Gillam (Chapter 5) demonstrates how people with dementia can communicate through song even when they are unable to make sense in sentences. She shows through her own clinical experience that people with dementia can use their non-verbal communication in music to express their inner spirit, and how rewarding this experience is for the facilitator. Killick and Allan (Chapter 10) have discussed how using photography, video and visual material offer powerful ways of communicating to those who find that language has become difficult. These media are not dependent on cognitive pathways and thus offer a special means to stimulate feelings, memories and imagination.

Art therapist, Pat Baines (Chapter 6), provides us with new insights as to how we can support people with dementia to express deep thoughts and feelings and also resolve difficult times in their lives through visual art. Baines supports the premise that all humans are creative beings and that people living with dementia also will communicate intimately and openly in a trusting environment. This author also provides practitioners with important research evidence supporting brain plasticity and brain reserve that can explain some of the unexpected and profound improvements seen in individuals with dementia who have opportunities to express themselves creatively.

Complementary therapies provide us with creative non-pharmacological alternatives in ways to physically and emotionally support people with dementia. Kirsten James covers a number of these approaches in her chapter (Chapter 7), with some practical ideas for safe implementation. She demonstrates how complementary therapies are person-led and represent creative ways of engaging individuals with dementia in a way that enables them to feel cared for and secure. James describes some of the science that supports the use of these therapies such as endorphin stimulation that can improve mood, promote relaxation, reduce pain and boost the immune system.

Telling each person's unique story is an art in itself, and Trisha Kotai-Ewers (Chapter 8) illustrates powerfully how a transformation in the person can occur through storytelling when facilitated both individually and in a group. She describes how this process can enable people to make sense of their present and past, because the stories represent the essence of our identity. Kotai-Ewers argues that giving people with dementia opportunities to tell their stories can not only help to prevent depression and anxiety, but also reduce the stigma of age and mental illness that are associated with older people with dementia. Storytelling provides opportunities to be listened to, to be understood and to express one's own truth; experiences that are too often lacking for those with dementia. This author's moving case studies show us that there is an important value in storytelling in exploring the meaning of changes that occur in the life of the person. Her practical strategies include approaches to understanding the creative language of people with dementia.

John Killick and Kate Allan (Chapter 10) explore new ground in their chapter on the use of photography and videography for whom language has become difficult. These media are not dependent on cognitive pathways and thus offer a special means to stimulate feelings, memories and imagination. These authors share their insights from projects and practical experience in a field that is emerging to have an important value and potentially wider application by health care professionals with people with dementia. This chapter includes the voices of people with dementia, who share their perceptions about what visual arts mean to them, and how this insight can enable health professionals and carers to find creative new ways to communicate.

Taking the time to know each individual is confirmed as essential by Pam Schweitzer in her chapter (Chapter 9)on innovative approaches to reminiscence. People with dementia will feel special, unique and valued as individuals if those who care for them know who they have been or who they are now, their stories, values, interests, likes and dislikes. This author stresses that listening to the person is vital to drawing them out, supporting their self-expression and enabling them to connect with others. She describes how appropriate multi-sensory stimuli can be closely matched to the individual's known background and life experience to trigger meaningful and personal memories.

Elizabeth MacKinlay (Chapter 11) shares her extensive research into how we affirm personhood and enable people with dementia to experience meaning in their lives. She highlights that to effectively facilitate well-being, we must include the spiritual dimension. Her recommendations include the importance of rituals (either religious or secular) to connect to meaning. She states that the search for meaning reaches to the core of human existence, which is the spiritual dimension. Trusted relationships can provide support to the person with dementia during this journey. MacKinlay recommends spiritual reminiscence with such relationships either individually or in small groups to explore meaning and spirituality.

John Killick and Kate Allan provide innovative ways to successful communication with those people who may have been given up on in the past, assuming they could no longer communicate. These authors discuss how important it is to be fully present for the person with dementia, especially at the end of their lives. They advise us to be in the moment, feeling less driven by our thoughts, more connected with our surroundings and to be at greater ease with time. They show us the value of being open to the person with dementia, to share not only what they are experiencing but what they are giving to us during the time we share with them. These authors take the view that all attempts at communication have meaning and have shared practical suggestions to connect with body language and take inspiration from the coma work of Mindell that uses close observation and mirroring of actions and sounds.

Conclusion

It is the editors' vision that this book will add a wider dimension to the traditional education of health professionals in order to give rise to a new understanding of the importance of person-centred creative approaches in dementia care. This book aims to encourage a shift to being open to new unchartered ground and the importance of bringing in professional creative artists and specialized practitioners to enhance a dementia care program.

Creativity is like electricity – it spreads with positive energy and ignites people. When combined with loving interactions the possibilities for creating improvement in people with dementia become real and exciting. A spectrum of limitless choices and options is available to all of us to select at will, and we can all learn to turn our imagination into reality. The readers will discover within this book that the arts and creative approaches have a far broader application than the traditional view of purely providing occupation.

References

Abraham, R. (2005). *When Words Have Lost Their Meaning: Alzheimer's Patients Communicate through Art*. New York: Praeger Publishers.

Cohen, G. D. (2000). *The Creative Age. Awakening Human Potential in the Second Half of Life*. New York: HarperCollins Publishers.

Csikszentmihalyi, M. (1992). *Flow: The Psychology of Happiness*. London, UK: Harper and Row.

Doidge, N. (2007). *The Brain That Changes Itself. Stories of Personal Triumph from the Frontiers of Brain Science*. Victoria, Australia: Scribe Publications Pty Ltd.

Estes, C. P. (1992). *Women Who Run with the Wolves*. London: Rider.

Gottlieb-Tanaka, D. (2006). *Creativity, Dementia and the Therapeutic Environment*. PhD Thesis. Vancouver, Canada: University of British Columbia.

Hannerman, B. T. (2006). Creativity with dementia patients. Can creativity and art stimulate dementia patients positively? *Geronotology*, 52, 59–65.

Kasayka, R. (2002). Introduction. In A. Innes & K. Hatfield (eds). *Healing Arts Therapies and Person-Centred Care*, London: Bradford Dementia Group Good Practice Guides, Jessica Kingsley Publishers.

Kitwood, T. (1993). Towards a theory of interpersonal care: the interpersonal process. *Ageing and Society*, 13, 51–67.

Kitwood, T. (1997). *Dementia Reconsidered. The Person Comes First*. Buckingham, UK: Oxford University Press.

Kitwood, T. (1998). *Dementia Care Mapping Course*, Bradford, UK: University of Bradford.

Kotai-Ewers, T. (2007). *Listen to the Talk of Us: People with Dementia Speak Out*. Shenton Park, WA: Alzheimer's Australia.

Lee, H. (2005, November). The great tapestry of life. *National Healthcare Journal*, 86.

Lee, H. (6 May 2006). *Weaving Memories and Dreams*. Paper presented at the Second International Conference on Creative Expression, Communication and Dementia, University of British Columbia, Vancouver, British Columbia, Canada.

Lee, H. (2007). Masters in Science (research). Thesis: *The impact of the Spark of Life Program on the personal and emotional wellbeing of people with dementia: carers' and families' perceptions*. Curtin University of Technology, Perth.

Lee, H. & Blades, K. (2007). *Connecting through creativity*. Presentation at the Hammond Care Group's Successful Ageing Conference, the Powerhouse Museum, University of Sydney, Sydney.

Power, A. (2010). *Dementia beyond Drugs*. Maryland, USA: Health Professionals Press Inc.

Power, A., Lee, H. & Verity, J. (2009) *Beyond Drugs in Dementia*. Plenary presentation. Dementia: Engaging Societies around the World. 24th Conference of Alzheimer's Disease International, Singapore.

Rogers, N. (1993). *The Creative Connection. Expressive Arts in Healing*. California: Science and Behaviour Books Inc.

Sachs, O. (2007). *Musicophelia. Tales of Music and the Brain.* London: Pan MacMillan Ltd.
Spitzer, P. (2008). LaughterBoss, Introducing a New Position in Aged Care. In B. Warren (ed.), *Using the Creative Arts in Therapy and Healthcare.* Sussex, UK: Routledge.
Taylor, R. (2009). Keynote presentation. Dementia: Engaging Societies Around the World. 24th Conference of Alzheimer's Disease International, Singapore.

1 Reigniting the human spirit

Jane Verity and Hilary Lee

Introduction

Every person is essentially many sparks of energy: 'sparks of life'. The spark represents the well-being of the human spirit. Ensuring a strong and healthy spirit is at the heart of the *Spark of Life* Philosophy, which offers a gentle, creative and celebratory approach to human relationships and communication. Although the philosophy was developed for dementia care, it has much wider application.

> Spirit is defined as the driving force that lies at the core of our being – the inner light that gives passion, meaning and purpose to our lives.
> (Jane Verity, 2008)

When a person loses those aspects of themselves that form their identity and give meaning and purpose in their life, the spark may become compromised and shine less brightly. It is as though the light has gone out of their eyes. However, this spark can again shine brightly once the person's spirit is reignited. The key to achieving this lies in the quality of the interaction that takes place between people. Once the communicator's energy changes, it has a profound effect on the quality of the outcome. When one's energy is focused on enriching the other person's life then it becomes possible to reignite the spirit.

The concept adds new depth to the traditional approach to dementia. A clear way to illustrate this is to use the analogy of an iceberg: one-tenth represents the visible part of the iceberg above the surface. Nine-tenths represent the invisible parts below the surface. For over 100 years, the traditional approach to dementia has focused on the one-tenth: on what is visible and observable, such as symptoms, behaviours, scans, mental test scores, diagnosis, prognosis and treatment. The *Spark of Life* Philosophy focuses on what is below the surface, the nine-tenths that are invisible and cannot be measured, such as the use of intuition, the need for love, the health of the human spirit, unmet emotional needs and the quality of energy transferred between people during any interaction.

It is in the realm below the surface that the root cause of many behavioural symptoms is found. By exploring what cannot be seen, measured or weighed, the philosophy enables us to discover solutions that dissolve issues and ignite the human spirit.

In dementia care, the *Spark of Life* Philosophy is implemented as a club program for people with dementia, a torchbearers program for selected staff members and a culture enrichment program for everyone connected with an organization. These programs will be defined and illustrated later in this chapter.

In this chapter, we introduce the reader to the *Spark of Life* Philosophy, its theoretical foundations and the evidence base including research findings and international best practise evaluations. The reader will also be introduced to guidelines, examples of excellence and our vision for the future.

Theoretical foundations

A clearer understanding of the scientific, psychological and philosophical background to this process can be found in the following four theoretical foundations which have most significantly influenced the development of the *Spark of Life* Philosophy.

1. Quantum physics
2. Occupational science
3. Person-centred care
4. Neurolinguistic programming (NLP)

1. Quantum physics

A *quantum* is defined as the smallest unit of light, electricity or other energy that can possibly exist (Chopra, 2001).

Through quantum physics, it is understood that anything in the world, no matter how solid it appears in its smallest entity, is vibrating energy. Quanta are involved in the energy transfer of an interaction.

Through quantum physics, Einstein was the first to introduce the concept of vibrating energy connecting all things in the universe (Bohm & Hiley, 1993). Einstein and his colleagues proved that everything around us is connected by unbounded quantum energy fields (Bohm, 1980; Bohm & Hiley, 1993). Every cell in our body 'eavesdrops' on the energy of our thoughts. The quality and state of our thoughts will determine the quality and state of our health (Chopra, 2009).

It is at this minute energetic level that the real cause and effect of human relationship and communication happens. Even an observer's energy can affect an outcome. Once a person has an awareness of the power of their energy, they can then choose to consciously bring the most positive energy to the interaction.

Quantum physics has influenced the *Spark of Life* Philosophy by:

- providing the scientific background behind the philosophy of igniting the human spirit. When the spirit is high it affects the thoughts, which in turn affects the health of both body and mind;
- offering the knowledge that everything is vibrating energy – thus the approach focuses on the energetic level of communication and interaction and the quality of energy transferred between two people;
- validating the body, mind and spirit connection; thereby showing why it is possible for this process to provide emotional, physical, mental and spiritual improvement.

2. Occupational science

Occupational Science is both a social science and a moral philosophy that enables people to regain lost skills and adapt back to normal life whether through learning new skills or adaptation through the environment. Hilary Lee (Dementia Care Australia, 2010)

The focus of occupational science is to enable independence with an emphasis on providing meaning in life. It is a whole person's approach focusing on the physical, social and psychological needs and amplifying a person's strengths and abilities.

Occupational science has influenced the *Spark of Life* Philosophy by:

* acknowledging the importance of focusing on a person's strengths and abilities, which is why the concept redefines a person's disabilities in terms of their abilities – such as redefining the term 'people who no longer communicate' to instead 'people who now communicate more through sounds, gestures and body language rather than through words and sentences';
* providing the science and moral duty to adapt our approach to suit individual needs, which is why the concept educates practitioners to continuously adapt their interaction and everything they do;
* providing the scientific basis for the *Spark of Life* Clubs (therapeutic group sessions) to be divided into 3 levels (of dementia) enabling all interactions to be adapted to best suit the needs of the individual members.

3. Person-centred care

Person-centred care represents a cultural change from management of the disease to care of the whole person. The late Professor Tom Kitwood laid the foundations for a new paradigm in dementia when he identified that, with the right attitude, it is possible to improve not only the mood and quality of life of people who have dementia but also their cognitive abilities. He considered that personhood remains intact; that the interpersonal environment has striking effects on a person with dementia and that there is potential for growth – rementia (Kitwood, 1997).

Person-centred care has influenced the *Spark of Life* Philosophy by:

* inspiring the development of an 'antidote' to the Malignant Social Psychology identified by Professor Tom Kitwood in

which 17 negative behaviours of people in the care environment were identified. The concept provides a detailed, practical and systematic method to transform those behaviours that undermine self-esteem and break the spirit into actions that lift the spirit and create opportunities for overall improvement and well-being.

4. Neurolinguistic programming (NLP)

N = Neuro = Brain
L = Linguistic = Language
P = Programming = Programming

NLP is a model of communication that describes how language is used to program our brain to achieve the highest possible results whilst ensuring that everyone's needs are regarded (ecology). It is the art and science of communication. Originally developed by Richard Bandler and John Grinder, NLP explains how information is processed. A core belief is that the internal representation made about the outside event is not necessarily the same as the event itself.

NLP has influenced the *Spark of Life* Philosophy by:

- looking for the underlying root cause of challenging behaviour;
- identifying the significance of preferred sensory channels in communication;
- such as visual, auditory and kinaesthetic;
- redefining negative, static labels to positive, workable opportunities such as from challenging behaviour to unmet need;
- providing communication tools to connect with people who have dementia;
- giving memory enhancement techniques based on neurological knowledge of how long-term memory is stimulated.

Evidence base

A number of studies have been undertaken on the *Spark of Life* Philosophy. There has been an extensive clinical application of

the approach internationally, which has provided much anecdotal data demonstrating that the program is effective in a
variety of situations and diverse cultures.

The following is a summary of some of the evidence col-
lated to date: A qualitative study using in-depth interviews
from Curtin University of Technology, Perth, Australia,
examined the perceptions of carers and families of the impact
of the *Spark of Life* Club Program on the personal and emotional well-being of people with dementia (Lee, 2007). The
club program is a therapeutic intervention designed to be used
in residential care and day centres that aims to address the
social, emotional, cultural and spiritual needs of people with
dementia.

Four main themes emerged from the data:

1 **Reigniting the human essence (the spirit)**
   The club members gained confidence, improved their
   social and communication skills, reengaged in life with
   vitality and renewed energy, demonstrated improvements
   in memory and were oriented to time, events and dates.
2 **Developing a sense of creativity**
   Club members were able to communicate in new ways
   through music, by expressing humour, being playful and
   telling 'prickly' or deeply emotional life stories to one
   another.
3 **Being in their shoes**
   Staff and family members perceived people with dementia
   in a new light, and recognized their potential for improvement and learning.
4 **Enabling success**
   The degree of success of the program was attributed to
   several factors: the personal qualities and attitude of
   staff, training for the whole care team, specific strategies
   used during the program such as the Lead by Following
   Method and the support and commitment of the facility
   management.

In conclusion, participation in the club program continues
to enable people with dementia to experience overall improvement. Even those who were thought lost to this world have

come out of their shell and reconnected with the world around them.

In 2008, a study by Gottlieb-Tanaka, Lee and Graf at the University of British Columbia, Canada, led to the development of the Creative Expressive Abilities Assessment (CEAA) Tool. The club program was selected as a quality creative expression program for observation in the study. The club members observed in this study scored highly in all domains of the CEAA tool, including memory, language, psychosocial skills, reasoning, expression of emotions and culture (Gottlieb-Tanaka, Lee & Graf, 2008).

In Wisconsin, USA, the club program has been endorsed as recommended best practice by the Wisconsin Adult Day Services Association (WASDA) and in a collaborative study between the Wisconsin Bureau of Aging and disability resources and the Wisconsin Office of Quality Assurance (Dementia Care Australia, 2010).

An International Best Practice Evaluation of the culture enrichment program is now being implemented in Australia, New Zealand and Canada. Initial findings provided in a report by Lee (2008), demonstrated that the culture enrichment program encourages flexibility and willingness to work beyond boundaries resulting in satisfied and energized teams and raised the standard of care.

A quality assurance report from Rockhampton in Queensland discusses the relationship between the reduction in falls and the *Spark of Life* Program (Quality Performance Systems, 2008). In July 2009, The *Spark of Life* Culture Enrichment Program was awarded the 2009/2010 IAHSA Excellence in Ageing Services Award for its whole systems approach and for being a model of innovation, creativity and excellence that also recognizes the importance of valuing the social capital of an organization. According to Christa Monkhouse, IAHSA and EAHSA Board Member, '*Spark of Life* was unanimously chosen because it has the potential to reverse the declinist view of dementia and ageing in general and to introduce an optimistic approach towards rementia and dementia rehabilitation' (Monkhouse, personal communication, 2010).

An evaluation at an aged care facility in Perth, Western Australia found that the culture enrichment program led to improvement in residents' function, well-being and social skills, with benefits in enriching the staff culture, which has seen the home become a preferred employer. In addition, the staff had been reinvigorated and new insights and skills were gained into how to cope with the challenges and stresses experienced in aged care. Positive outcomes were reported from the residents having participated in the club program and were demonstrated through the use of The Creative Expressive Abilities Assessment Tool and the Bradford Well-being Profile (The *Standard*, 2009).

As described above, the club program has been shown, through several studies as well as extensive clinical experience, to facilitate improvements in people with dementia. There are a number of possible neurological and biological reasons for this.

In her research, Lee (2007) discusses the links between enriched environments and plasticity in the brain, citing Kemperman and Gage (1999) and Schaffer and Gage (2004). Dr Norman Doidge (2007) defines neuroplasticity as the ability of the brain to change its structure with each activity it performs, perfecting its circuits to be better suited to the task at hand. Doidge's experience as a psychiatrist and researcher shows that the brain has the potential to heal itself in situations previously considered impossible.

Lee also argues, based on research from Charnetski and Brennan (2001), that the club members' experience of boosted self-esteem and confidence may have also enhanced their immune system. This notion is supported by Dr Ruth Cilento, author of *Age without Alzheimer's*, who states that it is the '*Spark of Life*' that alters the chemistry in the brain strengthening the immune system (Cilento, 2004).

Moreover, Dr Al Power in his book *Dementia beyond Drugs* (2010) observed that the impact of the *Spark of Life* Club Program facilitates 'rementia', meaning the reversal of the excess disability found in people with dementia when only a medical approach is used.

Examples of good practice

The **club program** is a therapeutic group intervention designed to be used in residential care and day centres that aims to address the social, emotional, cultural and spiritual needs of people with dementia. It is designed for people with all levels of dementia and is versatile in that it can be implemented with those who are bedridden and experiencing severe levels of dementia as well as being adapted to suit frail older people.

Case study

Ces had dementia for several years caused by Parkinson's disease and he was 'living in his own world'. He had not communicated with people around him for over 12 months and had been assessed as being beyond benefitting from participating in the club program. However, the decision was made to give Ces the opportunity to participate and he was invited to his first club session.

At first he sat with his eyes closed, appearing unreachable. Ces was then given the opportunity to choose between two musical instruments, a 'tapping' or a 'ringing' one. With gentle encouragement and unconditional regard, the facilitators persisted in a loving way providing the two choices in different ways with different levels of stimulation. Finally their efforts paid off, with Ces gradually coming out of his shell and murmuring his very first words in over 12 months, 'tapping one'.

He was invited to the whiteboard with a display of bright colourful musical notes and was encouraged to roll a giant dice with the same colours as the notes. He rolled the colour red and was encouraged to pick the red note. On the back of the note was the song: 'White Cliffs of Dover'. To bring the song alive, Ces was given an Australian army slouch hat and a mirror to see himself wearing the hat. Everyone including Ces then sang 'White Cliffs of Dover'.

The facilitator's patience was rewarded as Ces was brought back to the time he was serving in the Second World War. He began to reminisce about those horrendous experiences, talking in fluent sentences. Ces had come out of his shell and from that moment he 'chose' to be present in reality.

His wife Dell came in at the end of the session, moved to tears to see her Ces having 'come back'. In his wheelchair, he and Dell, sang and danced together. Ces's return to our reality lasted for three-and-a half years up until his death. He attended his last Spark of Life Club four days before he passed away and although his Parkinson's disease had affected his ability to speak, he was fully present with a sparkle in his eyes.

The torchbearer program is an educational program for selected staff members to keep the spark alight in their facility/

organization. It enables these staff members to grow the culture in their organization through focusing on creative ways to support their colleagues and amplify the positive. One of the strategies that torchbearers use to keep the spark ignited is to provide descriptive appreciation in various creative ways.

Over the years, torchbearers have come up with many ways of showing such spontaneous appreciation to their colleagues.

Case study

One team of Torchbearers wanted to appreciate their care manager who was extremely supportive so they wrote personal notes of appreciation on heart-shaped post-it notes and covered the entire door to her office in hearts; when she arrived she had a most unexpected heartwarming surprise. She kept all her heart notes in an envelope in her desk and took them out to read on tough days.

Another torchbearer group chose to honour one of their colleagues who was running late for their meeting and who they knew was feeling emotionally fragile. They too wrote descriptive appreciations on heart-shaped post-it notes. When their colleague arrived, they invited her to sit in the centre of the circle and one by one they took turns in reading out their appreciation, then giving her a 'heart attack' by sticking their heart on her in a genuine, but playful, way. She was overcome with positive emotions. Through her tears she thanked everyone and told how she often felt she was 'not good enough' but now she felt a whole person.

A team member, Joanna, had been going through a rough personal time and after a long absence returned to work but was insecure and withdrawn, keeping everyone at a distance. The torchbearers invited all their colleagues to write a note about what they truly appreciated about Joanna on a post-it note that was cut out in the shape of a balloon. They placed all the notes on a board and invited Joanna to a special afternoon tea where they presented the board of appreciations. Joanna was moved to tears, felt welcomed back into the workplace and began to reconnect with the group.

The culture enrichment program provides education and ongoing support to apply the philosophy across a whole organization. It involves everyone in a care facility from management and board members to all health care professionals, personal carers, volunteers and family members. The program works on the notion that all culture change happens from management level and ripples out to every area of the organization. In essence, it is about management empowering everyone to have a voice and tapping into the positive qualities of each person.

To facilitate such an empowerment shift, teams are taught to apply the principles of the *Spark of Life* Solution Circle – a culture enrichment tool.

Case study

A resident in a nursing home asked if they could have a dog. This request caused a myriad of objections, from, 'Who would pay the veterinarian bill, and the maintenance?' 'What about the allergies?' 'Who is going to clean up after the dog?' 'What about infection control?'

Instead of a decision being made at management level, the CEO invited the entire team to participate in a solution circle, where a round was conducted to identify all objections. These objections were then written up on a whiteboard and divided into four categories: one of cost, one of dog care plan, one of legislation and one of personnel.

The entire team then split into four groups, each addressing one of the four categories by working in a solution circle. At this stage, the entire focus of the group was devoted exclusively to identifying solutions. After 20 minutes, all four groups had successfully overcome their set of objections and experienced a heightened level of enthusiasm.

Everyone reconnected in the large circle and each group took turns in sharing its solution. After each group had shared, every person who had posted an objection in that particular category was asked if they felt the solution had satisfactorily met their objection. The result was that all objections were overcome. Two of the staff members even shared that they did not like dogs and had therefore objected. But after listening to everyone, they were now comfortable about a dog coming into the nursing home.

To everyone's surprise and delight they all realized that when they listened to each other's suggestions TOGETHER they could find the solutions to overcome any objection. As a team they decided that the next step would be to run a solution circle with the residents.

Practical guidance and direction

In the **club program**, staff, volunteers and students are carefully selected for their gentle and mature attitude to take on the roles of facilitators. They enable the club members to take the lead within the club meeting and encourage creative self-expression. Trust is built because facilitators ensure that every club member's contribution is validated and important, which in turn boosts their self-esteem and encourages them to contribute.

Name badges are an integral part of the club program and are worn by everyone, including club members, facilitators, visitors, volunteers or anyone else who participates in the club. The use of name badges encourages spontaneous interaction between club members and between club members and facilitators.

The club program applies a three-step rule which enables people with dementia to perform at his or her best so everyone can experience success.

Rule 1: Use one room that can be closed off from outside distractions.

Rule 2: Have at least two facilitators run the program.

Rule 3: Use three club levels enabling adaptation of the theme activities to suit the different abilities of people with dementia.

Another feature of the club program is the use of rituals, which provide a structure as well as familiarity and safety. These include Inviting ritual, Welcoming ritual, Beginning and Ending ritual.

Activities used in the club program are chosen specifically for their ability to encourage each individual club member to take the lead, to be creative and spontaneous, to have their self-esteem boosted and to express themselves freely.

The actual theme and the rituals are brought alive through creating ceremony, which means transforming ourselves and the environment into an extraordinary experience using music, scents, props and costumes.

One of the essential strategies used in the **torchbearer program** is descriptive appreciation. This provides a genuine and sincere way to say thank you that boosts another person's self-esteem.

To appreciate another person, it is necessary to engage both heart and mind for the experience to make a real difference. Here are two helpful steps to follow.

1. Clearly describe WHAT the other person has done or said that you wish to appreciate.
2. HOW it has made a difference to you or someone else.

An example could be: 'Thank you Gail for the way you greet me every day as I come in to work' (the WHAT) – 'you have no idea how much that means to me. I feel welcome and appreciated and that is a good way to start the day' (the HOW).

This strategy can also be successfully used with residents, their families, colleagues and your own family.

Using a circle to find creative solutions and resolve conflict has its roots in ancient, indigenous cultures where tribal elders would get together in a circle to decide on the laws of the tribe and to solve challenges. Today, circles are used successfully in many different ways, such as solving community issues and creating culture change such as the Eden Alternative.

In the **culture enrichment program** everyone is introduced to using the solution circle to overcome objections to new ideas. The following principles are helpful in ensuring a successful outcome.

All participants sit in a circle with one chair for each participant and no spare. It is recommended that a circle be no larger than eight to ten people. If any larger, it is better to break into smaller groups. The circle starts with one person volunteering to be the leader of that round. The leader invites two volunteers to come forward. Volunteer number 1 starts the round by being the first to respond or comment on the issue raised. Volunteer number 2 is the note taker. Only the person whose turn it is may talk.

When the turn comes to the leader, he or she shares their thoughts like everyone else. When the turn comes to the note taker, they pass the notepad and pen to the person who spoke before, and they write any points the note taker shares before handing back the notepad and pen. It can be a good idea to do two rounds even if no one passed in the first round to encourage everyone's ideas and input. The next step is to open up for discussion. A helpful strategy for listeners who are finding it hard to wait with a comment is to write their thoughts down so they are captured for when it is their turn.

In conclusion the solution circle is used to give everyone a voice in reaching creative and innovative solutions to culture enrichment challenges and objections (see example above in the section on good practice).

Conclusion and way forward

The *Spark of Life* Philosophy is about redefining what it means to have dementia and the possibilities for people with dementia when given new opportunities, while supported with love and compassion. *Spark of Life* has been successfully implemented in diverse cultures around the world and has the potential for broader application as an approach to the creative arts. Facilitators wanting to know more about how to access education about the philosophy or how to join this movement for social change in dementia care can visit www.dementiacareaustralia.com.

It is the vision of the authors of this chapter that a new dawn is emerging for people with dementia, a new future where the importance of keeping the spirit ignited is acknowledged as a priority. Applying the principles of the philosophy in what we do enables all of us – health care practitioners, students and family carers – to amplify the best of our human qualities, and enrich the culture of care. This is a vision of hope for people with dementia and all who support them. We conclude with Eleanor Roosevelt's wisdom:

> The future belongs to those who believe in the beauty of their dreams.

References

Bohm, D. (1980). *Wholeness and the Implicit Order*. Oxon., UK: Routledge and Kegan Paul.

Bohm, D. & Hiley, B. J. (1993). *The Undivided Universe. An Ontological Interpretation of Quantum Theory*. Oxon., UK: Routledge.

Charnetski, C. J. & Brennan, F. X. (2001). *Feeling Good Is Good for You. How Pleasure Can Boost Your Immune System and Lengthen Your Life.* New York: St. Martin's Press.

Chopra, D. (2001). *Perfect Health. The Complete Mind Body Guide.* North Sydney: Transworld Publishers, Random House Australia Pty Ltd.

Chopra, D. (2009). *Reinventing the Body, Resurrecting the Soul.* Chatham, UK: Rider, Ebury Publishing.

Cilento, R. (2004). *Age without Alzeheimer's*: Book One. Brisbane: Imprint Group.

Dementia Care Australia (2010). *Introduction to the Spark of Life Concept Module 1. Companion Workbook for the Spark of Life Certified Practitioner.* Mooroolbark, Victoria: Dementia Care Australia, p. 21.

Doidge, N. (2007). *The Brain That Changes Itself. Stories of Personal Triumph from the Frontiers of Brain Science.* Victoria, Australia: Scribe Publications Pty Ltd.

Gottlieb-Tanaka, D., Lee, H. & Graf, P. (2008). *The Creative-Expressive Abilities Assessment User Guide,* Vancouver, Canada: ArtScience Press.

Kempermann, G. & Gage, F. H. (1999). New nerve cells for the adult brain. *Scientific American,* 280(5), 38–43.

Kitwood, T. (1997). *Dementia Reconsidered. The Person Comes First.* Buckingham, UK. Oxford University Press.

Lee, H. (2007) Masters in Science (research). Thesis: *The impact of the Spark of Life program on the personal and emotional wellbeing of people with dementia: carer's and families perceptions.* Curtin University of Technology, Perth.

Lee, H. (2008). *Evaluation of the Spark of Life Culture Enrichment Program.* Report available on www.dementiacareaustralia.com, accessed on 1.12.10.

Power, A. (2010). *Dementia beyond Drugs.* Maryland, USA: Health Professional Press Inc.

Schaffer, D. & Gage, F. (2004). Neurogenesis and neuroadaptation. *Neuromolecular Medicine,* 5(1), 1–9.

The *Standard* (July 2009), *Spark of Life Wins International Recognition for Brightening Up Lives.* Parramatta, New South Wales: Aged Care Standards and Accreditation Agency Ltd., pp. 2–3.

Quality Performance Systems (2008). A Spark of Life Is Igniting Rockhampton Aged Care. 31, 4–7.

Verity, J. (2008). *The Spark of Life* Club Program. Educational manual and DVD set. Dementia Care Australia, Mooroolbark, Victoria.

Website link

www.dementiacareaustralia.com/index.php/library/research-findings.html, retrieved 19. 8.10.

2 The LaughterBoss™

Peter Spitzer

It is the job of the LaughterBoss, via open-heart surgery, to touch the soul and give it room to smile and laugh.

Peter Spitzer

Introduction

The LaughterBoss is a member of the health care team which has developed the creative skills to introduce humour and laughter into its facility.

LaughterBoss originates from the philosophy that laughter is the best medicine. The introduction of humour and laughter into older people and dementia care facilities assists staff to creatively enhance quality of life and psychosocial needs (McGuire & Boyd, 1993). The LaughterBoss is also well placed to help reduce staff stress and improve staff morale.

The LaughterBoss is a modern day equivalent of the court jester. It brings together the art of performance and health care and uses humour therapy as part of the facility's daily life. Ideal candidates for training are staff members who have intimate knowledge of residents and families as well as a thorough understanding of the environment and culture of the facility.

This chapter explores the training and introduction of the LaughterBoss into residential homes for older people.

Humour therapy, clowning and evidence-based medicine

Gelotology is the study of humour and its effects on the human body (Berk et al., 1989; Dillon, 1985; Fry, 1994; Fry

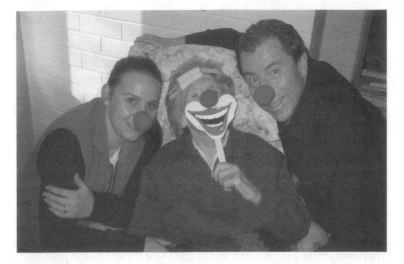

Figure 2.1   A LaughterBoss and Dr Spitzer with Madge, the Irish actress who refused to retire

et al., 1987; Gelkopf & Kreitler, 1996). The Association for Applied and Therapeutic Humor (AATH), founded in 1988, defines therapeutic humour as 'any intervention that promotes health and wellness by stimulating a playful discovery, expression, or appreciation of the absurdity or incongruity of life's situations. This intervention may enhance health or be used as a complimentary treatment…to facilitate healing or coping whether physical, emotional, cognitive, social or spiritual' (AATH, 2007).

Laughter affects the mind and the body. There are many reasons why laughter makes us feel good and a recent study has found that humour and laughter trigger the brain's reward centres (Mobbs et al., 2003). Other studies show respiratory and cardiovascular effects (Fry, 1977). Laughter stimulates respiration, relaxes arteries and improves blood flow as well as oxygen saturation of peripheral blood. After a transient rise there is a drop in blood pressure (Fry & Savin, 1988). Positive effects on hypertension and diabetes have been noted. A relaxation response is experienced after laughter. Laughter has been researched in the field of psychoneuroimmunology and studies have shown a drop in serum (cortisol) stress hormone (Berk et al., 1989), and enhancement of immune system functioning (Dillon et al., 1985–1986). Laughter is also studied in the field of Positive Psychology (Snyder & Lopez, 2006) and positive effects on performance, mood, optimism, anxiety and depression have been observed. Enhanced communication and positive association with emotional stability are also noted. Laughter has also been used as a non-pharmacological tool to help manage pain.

Clowning has a long history of being an art form that invites play, interaction and above all laughter (Otto, 2001). On the front page of the September 1908 issue of *Le Petit Journal* there is a drawing of two clowns working their craft in a London children's hospital ward. In Turkey, several centuries ago, the Dervishes who were responsible for the well-being of their patients, first fed the body and then used their performance skills to feed the soul. More recently, hospital clowning has become established in many countries with palpable benefits to patients, families and staff.

The court jester (or fool) (Otto, 2001) was a particular type of clown associated with the Middle Ages. In those days they were thought of as special cases that God had touched with a childlike madness. They wore bright, motley patterned costumes and floppy cloth hats with three points each having a jingle bell at the end. They also carried a mock sceptre.

"Above all he used humor, whether in the form of wit, puns, riddles, doggerel verse, songs, capering antics or nonsensical babble, and jesters were usually also musical or poetic or acrobatic, and sometimes all three." (Otto, 2001)

The tradition of court jesters lasted about 400 years and they worked in the royal courts of Europe, the Middle East and Asia.

Patch Adams as a young doctor in the 1970s, began clowning for hospital patients. Big Apple Circus established the Clown Care Unit in New York City in 1987 and was the first structured hospital clown program with frequent and regular visits to host hospitals.

There are many hospital clowning programs around the world where hospital clowns work in partnership with other health care providers. Professionalism of the hospital clowns and the programs they deliver are a high priority with regular training programs and quality assurance reviews. Clowning in hospitals addresses the psychosocial needs of patients as well as the facility as a whole.

There are many published studies on the effects of humour and laughter in aged care and a small number is referenced here (Barrick et al., 1990; Dean, 1997; Fox, 1990; Fry, 1986; Hulse, 1994; McGuire et al., 1992; McGuire et al., 1993; Richmond, 1995; Simon, 1988; Williams, 1986).

It is acknowledged that care of the growing elder population is under increasing pressure. In Australia, over 150,000 people live in Residential Aged Care Facilities (RACFs) with half in high-level RACFs (nursing homes) and half in low- level RACFs (hostels) (Australian Institute of Health Welfare, 2007). In 2005–2006, $7.5 billion of recurrent government funding was spent on RACFs. Rates of dementia are high affecting over 70% of people in nursing homes and over 25% of those in hostel care. The quality of life in RACFs varies considerably. Levels of depression have been reported as 40% in high-level care and 25% in low-level care (Snowdon & Fleming, 2008). More than 90% of people with dementia will have at least one behavioural or psychological symptom (Brodaty et al., 2001). Behavioural disturbances are accompanied by high stress levels amongst staff (Brodaty et al., 2003) and average annual staff turnover rates are high with 20% for nurses and 25% for assistants in nursing (Richardson & Martin, 2004).

Humour as non-pharmacological therapy in the older person

Humour tends to stay with the person very late into dementia. Older persons who have a better sense of humour and use humour as a coping mechanism are more likely to live longer (Svebak et al., 2006), age well (Solomon, 1996) and be more satisfied with their physical health and life in general (Celso et al., 2003). While older adults may have poorer comprehension of humour than younger persons as a result of age related cognitive decline, they have similar levels of enjoyment when they do find something humorous (Mak & Carpenter, 2007; Shammi & Stuss, 2003). It has long been appreciated that there is great inter-individual variation in what is considered humorous (Eysenck, 1943), and some age-differences on humour 'tests' may be due to cohort effects. Interviews with nursing-home residents have found that they seldom experience humour in RACFs (Isola & Astedt-Kurki, 1997). This may be because RACFs offer few opportunities to experience humour and/or because residents do not always consider mainstream delivery of humour (e.g. television) funny.

Few studies have evaluated the efficacy of humour therapy in institutionalized older persons. Four of the five studies showed some benefit, although they were limited by small sample sizes, relatively low quality methodology and lack of flexibility in matching humour to residents' capabilities (two studies only). A study (n = 21) of four clown sessions evaluated using a modified dementia care mapping protocol found an overall increase in positive behaviours and decrease in negative behaviours during the sessions in persons with severe dementia (Thomson, 2005). A controlled study (n = 61) found that five sessions of comical singing and dancing were associated with decreased self-rated anxiety and depression in older residents (Houston et al., 1998). Residents (n = 87) who watched humorous movies 3 times a week for 12 weeks showed decreased negative affect over time compared to controls who received usual care(Boyd & McGuire, 1996). Fortnightly group humour therapy for psychiatric inpatients with Alzheimer's disease or late-life depression did not improve quality of life compared to standard pharmacotherapy (n = 20) (Walter et al., 2007). Residents (n = 27) who watched recordings of humorous storytelling weekly for 12 weeks reported improved quality of life compared to those who watched conventional television or usual care (Ronnberg, 1998).

The recent emergence of clowning in RACFs

Several organizations deliver (modified) clowning programs to RACFs. These include

- Big Apple Circus Clown Care Unit Vaudeville Caravan, USA,
- Hearts & Minds Elderflowers, Scotland,
- Fools for Health Family Clowns, Canada,
- Humour Foundation ElderClowns, Australia.

Although these programs operate independently, a number of common themes have emerged and these include: avoiding the hospital/doctor persona of the performer as used in hospitals, avoiding stethoscopes and medical schticks, more detailed briefing by staff, sensitive tailored interactions based on individual needs, flexibility in delivering multiple art forms and toning down of costumes and characters. All performers continue wearing the red nose.

Big Apple Circus Clown Care Unit Vaudeville Caravan, USA

Big Apple Circus' *Vaudeville Caravan* was conceived in 2001 (Chicago, USA) as a logical outgrowth of Clown Care and the idea that laughter and delight have a place in residential nursing care facilities. Recognizing that theatre and circus arts have a universal appeal that make them effective in reaching people no matter their age or background, the *Vaudeville Caravan* approach emphasizes highly interactive, individualized interactions. By incorporating a repertoire of recognizable songs from the seniors' era, puppetry, dance and magic, these artists empower seniors to participate in the action and express positive emotions, thereby creating a community among residents and staff and counteracting the loneliness and isolation that can be part of life in RACFs.

Hearts & Minds Elderflowers, Scotland

A qualitative evaluation reviewed the social, emotional and psychological impact of their program in RACFs. Positive changes were observed on people with dementia, staff and families.

Fools for Health Familial-Clowns, Canada

Professor Bernie Warren in his article 'I remember you ... Who's your friend?' The Work of Fool's for Health's Familial-Clowns with Seniors with Dementia ('Down Memory Lane' project funded by The Ontario Trillium Foundation) discusses strategies used by the Familial-Clowns (Ontario, Canada) to return power to individuals who have little control over their life. These strategies are delivered by character-based clowns who use little or no stage make-up. This sets them apart from 'circus clowns' who need to wear bright and loud make-up and costume so as to be seen when working under the big top. This highly stylized face painting is unnecessary and can elicit adverse reaction when working in RACFs.

Again, positive changes were noted. Also included in the paper is discussion on the value of the smile and the use of creativity and imagination.

The Humour Foundation was co-founded by the author in 1997. This national charity is dedicated to promoting the health benefits of humour. The core project, the Clown Doctors™, has been delivering humour therapy to paediatric hospitals, general hospitals and palliative care facilities since then. Clown Doctors are professional performers trained to work in hospital settings.

Visits to residential aged care facilities (have been irregular and has limited the impact and connection with everyone in the facility. The comment 'Why don't you come more often?' signalled an inadequately met need.

The Foundation's financial constraints meant that the increasing demand for Clown Doctors to visit aged care facilities could not be met. As a result, the author developed the LaughterBoss concept. In this initiative, staff members were taught humour intervention skills which they delivered on a regular and opportunistic basis.

The LaughterBoss model was introduced at *The First National Conference on Depression in Aged Care: 'Challenging Depression in Aged Care'* at the University of New South Wales, Sydney, Australia, June 2003.

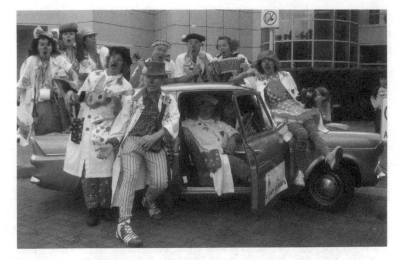

Figure 2.2   Nothing ever surprises Clown Doctors

Who and what is the LaughterBoss?

The LaughterBoss is a modern day equivalent of the court jester. The main role of the LaughterBoss is to bring play, humour and laughter into the facility.

While the main focus of the LaughterBoss is on the residents, a positive impact on staff, visitors and the general community has been reported. The LaughterBoss can reduce staff stress and improve morale as well as assist staff to enhance quality of life, reduce depression and meet psychosocial needs of people with dementia. This is done through assisting communication, increased support, giving residents cognitive control, providing positive diversion and generally increasing the 'smileage' factor.

Ideal candidates for LaughterBoss training are facility staff members who have an intimate knowledge of the people (residents, staff and families) and a thorough understanding of the environment and culture of the facility. The LaughterBoss position is added onto the 'day job' of the staff member. This not only reduces costs but also addresses and enhances recommended multifaceted interventions.

Training doesn't make the LaughterBoss a professional performer, but they do emerge as a new identity in the facility. They should be easily recognizable and available to do their work at a moment's notice as the need arises. They also lead the way in introducing themes, special days and events.

LaughterBoss training

The initial training is a full-day experiential program.

A. Selection

Applicants often self-select and are motivated to attend training. They must have the acknowledgement and support of senior staff and management. The philosophy of the LaughterBoss must be a good fit with the philosophy of the RACF. Applicants come from nursing and allied health care staff. Often, training grants cover the cost of training.

Group size is limited to 20–30 people.

B. Course materials and teaching aids

Each trainee receives a resource pack. It contains information on the Humour Foundation Clown Doctor program that opens discussion on introducing new models into the health care setting. There is a paper on the LaughterBoss written by the author, a summary of therapeutic effects of laughter, review of laughing at vs. laughing with someone, humour resources, a list of creative ideas, taking steps towards an optimistic state of mind and a paper on the health benefits of optimism, a nursing journal paper on the 'Use of humour in Patient Care', a paper on 'The Therapeutic Power of Humor - Brief Article' and an academic and therapeutic reference list on Humour and Gerontology.

Humour resources and creative ideas give busy health care professionals a practical summary of what material is available, how it can be used as an intervention and where it can be sourced. This includes reading materials and (local) Internet access.

The scientific material and video clips are delivered using a data projector. One or two tables are used to hold reference books and materials as well as a variety of props.

Information on both psychological and physical benefits of laughter gives scientific evidence and helps underpin the validity of LaughterBoss.

C. Training content

Training brings a number of elements together by

(a) introducing the science behind the 'laughter is the best medicine' quote;
(b) exploring the 'Art of Medicine' and how to introduce humour and play;
(c) stimulating creativity and developing new skills;
(d) networking between like-minded health care professionals.

Training content

Session 1 includes: pre-training questionnaire, introduction to the LaughterBoss concept and introduction to each participant, group activities to have some fun and play with each other, introduction to the Humour Foundation Clown Doctor program, the science and psychoneuroimmunology underpinning laughter and humour, video clips and stories from the coal-face. Video clips, when available, give visual cues to laughter/play interactions. Photos are also used and give similar cues. Both open the door to deliver stories from the coal-face. Stories are a very important way of translating the theory to reality.

Session 2 includes: group play, developing a new view of the aged care space, introduction to the play basket, the humour notice board and resource material, brainstorming in groups of three on creative ways to humour one's self, residents and staff.

Group play includes a number of exercises that stimulate play. This is valuable experientially to balance the intellectual activities. Group plays show the value of brief interventions and are a good way of linking the participants.

Group plays are introduced in all the sessions. There are many appropriate group plays available. A good resource is *Playfair* (Matt Weinstein and Joel Goodman, Impact Publishers).

The play basket is in itself a play resource. A basket, strategically placed, can have a variety of colourful props such as scarves, wigs, hats, lightweight balls and so on, ready to be used at a moment's notice. Local businesses and community groups can connect with the facility by donating equipment. The humour notice board is also strategically placed. It invites humour. Residents, families and staff can add jokes/ humour articles/photos. The LaughterBoss maintains and supervises this space.

Resource material can be donated or made by the local community. This includes materials for the play basket as well as items such as puppets and balloons.

The brainstorming exercise is a way of including others in creative thought and expression. This is a safe and non-judgemental exercise in lateral thinking.

A selection of books on humour is on display throughout the day. Included is *The Best Friends Book of Alzheimer's Activities* (Bell, et al.,

Session 3 includes: more group play, using props as communication tools, using Polaroid and photography, examples of brief humour interventions, humour during entry and exit, introducing love heart tennis as an example of fun play that can incorporate residents, staff and family. It is engaging and uses hand-eye coordination and is more suited to people with a milder form of dementia.

A variety of props can be used to induce play, laughter and enhanced communication. These are on display and the 'schtick' is shown. Colourful, close-up magic often works well. Puppets also work well. Participants can experiment and play with the props during breaks in the training.

Given the busy-ness of the day, brief improvisations/ interventions make a difference, make sense and are achievable during a busy shift. These are shown and discussed. For instance, it may be possible for the resident to team up with the LaughterBoss to play a 'trick' on the family.

Entry and exit to the facility, the staff room, the dining room, the resident's living space are areas where the LaughterBoss can trip over themselves literally – a way of acknowledging human frailty even in the staff. This is theatre 'on the go'; this is brief intervention; this invites reaction and comment; this is play.

Session 4 includes: planning and introducing themes, exploring fun musical opportunities, aligning play to the resident's history, exploring the possibilities of the humour/play cart and the potential to connect with the broader community, different ways of being funny on excursions, dealing with dementia, question and answer segment and post-training questionnaire.

Additional comments on training

Themes for the day, the week, the month and a variety of special occasions are explored. For example, how does the LaughterBoss make Funny Fridays happen? Ways of engaging residents, their families and staff are discussed.

Photo opportunities can easily find their way to the residential or local newspaper. The message is that RACFs are part of the community.

A variety of musical/fun opportunities are explored. There are a variety of ways of forming an 'instant band'. The humour cart is, like the humour basket and the humour notice board, another opportunity of introducing play. The medication trolley brings medicine. The humour trolley brings play. This can have props as in the humour basket as well as props like the

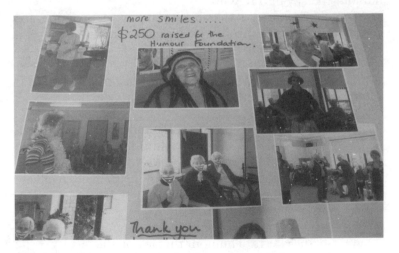

Figure 2.3   Raising smiles for the Humour Foundation

Polaroids, puppets, magic and balloons. These can be sourced from local community, schools and businesses – again linking the facility with the broader community.

Throughout the four sessions participants experience the Massage Train. This massage activity connects the group in a quick, enjoyable and light-hearted way. This activity can be used during staff handover/shift change. Anytime really. Each participant receives a colourful completion of training LaughterBoss certificate and usually a 'graduation' photograph is taken.

A pilot survey of LaughterBoss training for Northern Sydney Central Coast Health was conducted by Central Coast Research and Evaluation in 2005 – Gelotology in Gerontology: Integrating Humour Therapy into Dementia Care. LaughterBosses also provided anecdotal feedback that their humour interventions result in improvement in the quality of life of residents and staff morale.

Introducing a sustainable way forward for humour therapy in RACFs

Where specially trained professional performers are not able to be present, the LaughterBoss model is one way of introducing humour therapy into RACFs.

Maintaining humour therapy, upskilling, networking and continuation of training has been problematic especially for the isolated LaughterBoss.

SMILE study: researching a new humour therapy intervention model that builds on LaughterBoss

A landmark three-year prospective study has commenced in 2009. The SMILE (Sydney Multisite Intervention of LaughterBosses and ElderClowns) study, funded by NHMRC, is a clustered randomized trial of humour therapy involving approximately 400 people from 36 RACF units.

The aims of the SMILE study are to

• evaluate the effects of humour therapy on the quality of life of residents in RACFs;

- evaluate the effects of humour therapy on the level of mood and behavioural disturbance;
- evaluate the effects of humour therapy on staff burnout and turnover within the RACFs;
- determine the sustainability of the effects of the intervention;
- evaluate the costs and benefits of the intervention.

Whilst researching the effects of humour therapy, the modelling of the presentation of humour therapy has been reviewed and issues of sustainability and costs have been considered.

In this new model, an ElderClown will work together with a LaughterBoss hence addressing both of the above-mentioned issues in a practical way.

The ElderClown in the new model

Ideally, the ElderClown visits once a week and interacts with the residents as a group and individually with those for whom consent is available. The performer will develop a working partnership with the LaughterBoss and make connection with residents' families whenever possible.

The ElderClown is responsible for continuing to teach basic clowning skills as well as being a mentor to the LaughterBoss.

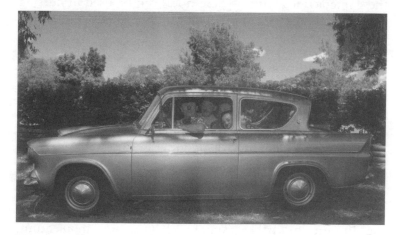

Figure 2.4 ElderClowns driving to work/play

ElderClowns are chosen from the ranks of working Clown Doctors from the Humour Foundation and receive additional training and experience in an aged care setting. ElderClowns are skilled professional performers auditioned, trained and experienced in clowning in care settings where people have different levels of physical, emotional and cognitive abilities and needs. ElderClowns are in part inspired by the Scottish Elderflowers program for persons with severe dementia in residential care.

The ElderClown, working with the LaughterBoss, play off each other non-threateningly while building rapport and trust with residents within and across visits. Humour therapy uses techniques such as storytelling, mime, song, magic and slapstick. The ElderClown is an improviser who uses the LaughterBoss to help gather information regarding the residents' abilities, previous history and interests. They then use their own experience and intuition to create tailored interactions, or 'plays' that better connect with the resident. For people with dementia these plays may allow them to act out of old scripts from their past – for example, a lady who had worked in a haberdashery store for a year may engage with an ElderClown comically pretending to lose and need to buy a replacement button. The ElderClown and LaughterBoss keep notes after each visit to facilitate the continued development of these interactions across. These notes can be used in nursing and medical reviews and may be of benefit in case of management reviews.

The LaughterBoss in the new model

The LaughterBoss will receive weekly input from visiting ElderClown as they work together. During the rest of the week the LaughterBoss works alone implementing new humour therapy interventions and/or building on interventions initiated by the ElderClown.

Every three months, booster, half-day training sessions for LaughterBosses and ElderClowns will allow refinement of skills as well as program review and continuing networking. In order to further promote self-sustaining momentum,

LaughterBosses will be encouraged to support and network with each other via email and telephone. LaughterBosses will be provided with some basic props to use in their plays and a small budget can be allocated to purchase props appropriate for the residents in their units.

How ElderClowns and LaughterBosses work together

> People with dementia seem to be more feeling than think-ing. Their language seems to be more symbolic than realistic. Not talking about what's in the words but what is behind the words.
>
> *John Killick*

On arrival at the RACF, the ElderClown meets with the LaughterBoss before starting their rounds. This time is used to discuss the profile and get an update of the resident with demen-tia they will be visiting. Entries about humour therapy interven-tions made in the resident's notes will also be reviewed. Choice of plays, music, costuming and so on, will be discussed.

In general, during the intervention, the ElderClown will be the principal performer with the LaughterBoss assisting and joining in the interaction as appropriate. There is opportunity for the LaughterBoss to take the lead role.

Debriefing, including note taking, takes place at the end of the intervention. Concepts for taking the humour therapy forward for the next week are proposed.

Pairing the ElderClown and LaughterBoss has multiple benefits:

* For the LaughterBoss, this will reinforce and augment their humour training, and give them ideas to try when the ElderClown is not present.
* For the ElderClown, they will be working with a staff member who knows the residents well and whom the resi-dents trust, facilitating building of a relationship with the ElderClown.
* For the resident, it means that the ElderClown interven-tions are sustained by the LaughterBoss.

LaughterBoss' Assistant

Some people with dementia have noticeable humour-related personality and skills. With due consideration and consent, they can take on the role of the LaughterBoss' Assistant and indeed give (supervised) assistance to the LaughterBoss.

Utilizing existing skills can sit next to learning and teaching new schticks.

Some LaughterBoss stories

Story 1

The Diversional Therapist was also the LaughterBoss at a hostel and nursing-home complex. Some people had mild dementia. She planned a special outing into the nearby town in the facility bus. Just for this outing, only people dressed funny could come along. The excitement in the facility was palpable for weeks prior to the event. People contacted family and friends for that right piece of clothing/hat/shoes/scarves. Make-up came out and was tested. The hairdresser was booked out. The energy level in the bus rose. People were animated. There was talk and laughter long after the event was over.

Story 2

The LaughterBoss was performing a juggle and magic routine for a person. She said that the routine was done in travelling circus shows in the 1930s. 'No' she was told by a seemingly distressed person. 'You've got it wrong. It was done like this!' and the LaughterBoss was told how it should be done properly.

This was no adverse reaction. It was the first time the person had spoken for weeks! That person not only continued talking but was also delighted to find a new situation in her life – as the LaughterBoss's Assistant.

Story 3

A Polaroid (or digital) camera can be used at a moment's notice when a photo opportunity presents itself. The process of getting ready can involve a story. This can take a minute or extend to several moments as everyone gets ready to be photographed. Polaroids are preferred as they give an immediate result. They can be left with the resident. Staff, family and friends usually make comments and this stimulates communication, connection and story telling.

At the beginning of the chapter, the photo 'With Madge – the Irish actress who never retired' is an example of the value of a photo opportunity. The photo has been enlarged and now has a cherished place in the family home.

Conclusion

It is predicted that by 2020 aged care service costs in Australia will rise from AUD 7 billion to AUD 12 billion (The Myer Foundation, 2002). The residential aged care sector struggles to maintain and improve quality of life of residents while operating within fiscal restraints and dealing with staff shortages, high staff turnover and increasing demands from consumers (Braithwaite, 2001).

SMILE is the first large-scale study of humour therapy anywhere in the world. SMILE uses a rigorous methodology to test an innovative intervention to make a positive impact in RACFs. If the use of humour therapy were to become

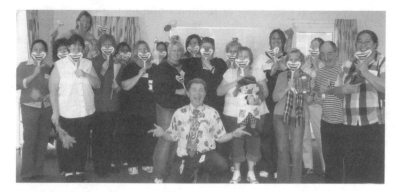

Figure 2.5   LaughterBoss graduation photo

widespread, the lives of thousands of older people, residing in homes for older people in Australia and around the world, could be improved.

Humour therapy, whilst specialized in its integration into RACFs, is not a stand-alone approach. It relies on the presence of excellence of philosophy and care in the RACF. The value of humour for people with dementia is acknowledged. Connecting professional performers, staff and people with dementia is a creative possibility that can open the heart and soul to the value of humour.

The LaughterBoss has a pivotal role in bringing about this positive change.

References

The Association for Applied and Therapeutic Humor (2007). www.aath.com, accessed on 9 Jan 2011.

Australian Institute of Health Welfare.

Barrick, A. L., Hutchinson, R. L. & Deckers, L. H. (1990). Humor, aggression and ageing. *Gerontologist*, 30(5), 675–678.

Bell, V., Troxel, D., Cox, T., Hamon, R. (2004). *The Best Friends Book of Alzheimer's Activities, Volume one.* USA, Health Professionals Press.

Berk, L. S., Tan, S. A., Fry, W. F., Napier, B. J., Lee, J. W., Hubbard, R. W., Lewis, J. E. & Eby, W. C. (1989). Neuroendocrine and stress hormone changes during mirthful laughter. *American Journal of the Medical Sciences*, 298(6), 390–396.

Boyd, R. & McGuire, F. (1996). The efficacy of humor in improving psychological well-being of residents of long term care facilities. *Journal of Leisurability*, 23 (4), 26–38.

Braithwaite, J. (2001). The challenge of regulating care for older people in Australia. *British Medical Journal.* 323: 443–6.

Brodaty, H., Draper, B. & Low, L- F. (2001). Psychosis, depression and behavioural disturbances in Sydney nursing home residents: prevalence and predictors. *International Journal of Geriatric Psychiatry*, 16(5), 504–512.

Brodaty, H., Draper, B. & Low, L- F. (2003). Nursing home staff attitudes towards residents with dementia: strain and satisfaction with work. *Journal of Advanced Nursing*, 44(6), 583–590.

Celso, B. G., Ebener, D. J. & Burkhead, E. J. (2003). Humor and aging well: a laughing matter or a matter of laughing? *Aging and Mental Health*, 7(6), 438.

Dean, R. A. (1997). Humor and laughter in palliative care. *Journal of Palliative Care,* 13(1), 34–39.

Dillon, K. M., Minchoff, B. & Baker, K. H. (1985–1986). Positive emotional states and enhancement of the immune system. *International Journal of Psychiatry,* 15(1), 13–18.

Evaluation of Hearts and Minds Clowndoctors and Elderflowers Programmes.Blake Stevenson Executive Summary, July 2007. www.bigapplecircus.org/community/vaudeville-caravan.aspx; www.heartsminds.org.uk; http://web2.uwindsor.ca/fools_for_ health/index.html; www.humourfoundation.com.au, accessed on 9 Jan 2011.

Eysenck, H. J. (1943). An experimental analysis of five tests of 'appreciation of humor'. *Educational and Psychological Measurement,* 3(1), 190.

Fox, K. (1990). Laugh it off: the effects of humor on the well-being of the older adult. *Journal of Gerontological Nursing,* 16(12), 11–16.

Fry, W. (1997). The respiratory components of mirthful laughter. *Journal of Biological Psychology,* 9, 39–50.

Fry, W. F. (1986). Humor, Physiology and the Ageing Process. *Humor and Ageing* (pp. 81–98). Orlando, FL: Academic Press.

Fry, W. F. (1994). The biology of humor. *HUMOR: International Journal of Humor Research,* 7(2), 111–126.

Fry, W. F. (1997). The respiratory components of mirthful laughter. *Journal of Biological Psychology,* 9, 39–50.

Fry, W. & Savin, W. (1988). Mirthful laughter and blood pressure. *Humor: International Journal of Humor Research,* 1, 49–62.

Fry, W. F. & Salameh. (1987). *Handbook of Humor and Psychotherapy: Advances in the Clinical Use of Humor.* Sarasota, FL: Professional Resource Exchange.

Goodman, J. & Weinstein, M. (1980). *PlayFair: Everyone's Guide to Noncompetitive Play.* San Luis Obispo, CA: Impact Publishers.

Gelkopf, M. & Kreitler, S. (1996). Is humor only fun, an alternative cure or magic? The cognitive therapeutic potential of humor. *Journal of Cognitive Psychotherapy: An International Quarterly,*10(4), 235–254.

Hammond Care Group. www.hammond.com.au/dsdc/conferences. php?conference=2003, accessed on 9 Jan 2011.

http://www.aag.asn.au/filelib/NSW_NOTES_May_2006.pdf - page 3; Gelotology in Gerontology: Integrating Humour Therapy into Dementia Care.

Houston, D. M., McKee, K. L., Carroll, L. et al. (1998). Using humor to promote psychological wellbeing in residential homes for older people. *Aging and Mental Health* ISSN 1360-7863, Online ISSN: 1364-6915, 2(4), 328.

Hulse, J. R. (1994). Humor: a nursing intervention for the elderly. *Geriatric Nursing*, 15(2), 88–90.

Hunter (Patch) Adams. www.patchadams.org, accessed on 9 Jan 2011.

Isola, A. & Astedt-Kurki, P. (1997). Humour as experienced by patients and nurses in aged nursing in Finland. *International Journal of Nursing Practice*, 3(1), 29.

Kelly, J. R. (ed.) (1993). *Activity and Aging: Staying Involved in Later Life*. Newbury Park, CA: Sage. pp. 164–173.

Killick, J. Reflecting on the work of the Elderflower project of the Hearts & Minds charity, Scotland.

Mak, W. & Carpenter, B. D. (2007). Humor comprehension in older adults. *Journal of the International Neuropsychological Society*, 13(04), 606.

McGuire, F. A. & Boyd, R. K. (1992). The Role of Humor in Enhancing the Quality of Later Life. In J. R. Kelly (ed.), *Activity and Aging*, 17(1), pp. 1–96.

McGuire, F. A., Boyd, R. K. & James, A. (1992). Therapeutic humor with the elderly. *Activities, Adaptations and Aging*, 17(1), 1–96.

McGuire, F. A. & Boyd, R. K. (1993). The Role of Humour in Enhancing the Quality of Later Life. *Activity & Aging: Staying Involved in Later Life*. Newbury Park, CA: Sage pp. 164–173.

Mobbs, D., Greicius, M. D., Abdel-Azim, E., Menon, V. & Reiss, A. L. (2003). Humor modulates the mesolimbic reward centres. *Neuron*, 40, 1041–1048.

National Health & Medical Research Council, Australian Government. Project Grant: 568787. http://www.nhmrc.gov.au/, accessed on 9 Jan 2011.

Otto, B. K. (2001). *Fools Are Everywhere: The Court Jester around the World*. Chicago: University of Chicago Press.

Richardson, S. & Martin, B. (2004). *The Care of Older Australians – A Picture of Residential Aged Care Workforce*. Adelaide: The National Institute of Labour Studies, Flinders University.

Richmond, J. (1995). The lifesaving function of humor with the depressed and suicidal elderly. *The Gerontologist*, 35(2), 271–273.

Ronnberg, L. (1998). Quality of life in nursing-home residents: an intervention study of the effect of mental stimulation through an audiovisual programme. *Age Ageing*, 27(3), 393.

Shammi, P. & Stuss, D. J. (2003). The effects of normal aging on humor appreciation. *Journal of the International Neuropsychological Society*, 9, 855.

Simon, J. J. (1988). Humor and the older adult: implications for nursing. *Journal of Advanced Nursing Practice*, 13, 441–446.

Snowdon, J. & Fleming, R. (2008). Recognising depression residential facilities: an Australian challenge. *International Journal of Geriatric Psychiatry*, 23(3), 295–300.

Snyder, C. R. & Lopez, S. J. (2006). *Positive Psychology: The Science and Practical Explorations of Human Strengths*. London: Sage.

Solomon, J. C. Humor and Aging Well. A Laughing Matter or a Matter of Laughing? *American Behavioral Scientist*. January 1996 39: 249–271.

Svebak, S., Kristoffersen, B. & Aasarod, K. (2006). Sense of humor and survival among a county cohort of patients with end-stage renal failure: a two-year prospective study. *International Journal of Psychiatry in Medicine*, 36(3), 269.

The Myer Foundation. 2020: A Vision for Aged Care in Australia.

Thomson, R. (2005). NHS Borders Psychological Services (Nov), 3.

Walter, W., Haani, B., Haug, M., Amrhein, I., Krebs-Roubicek, E., Müller-Spahn, F. & Savaskan, E. (2007). Humour therapy in patients with late-life depression or Alzheimer's disease: a pilot study. *International Journal of Geriatric Psychiatry*, 22, 77.

Williams, H. (1986). Humor and healing: therapeutic effects in geriatrics, *Gerontion*, 1(3), 14–17.

3 Dramatherapy and dementia care

Joanna Jaaniste

> Growing old is one of the ways the soul nudges itself into attention to the spiritual aspect of life.
>
> *Thomas Moore*

In every old person, there is a 'nudge' towards spiritual aware-ness – even an element of mysticism. It is important therefore that we recognize and honour these aspects and help older people have a creative and fulfilling final phase in their lives. Often in our society, people are 'socially dead' long before they are physically dead (Langley, 1987). It is essential that elderly people are respected in the way they are cared for and housed, though this is not always the case (Kitwood, 1997). People with dementia are doubly marginalized because of their illness and old age. It is painful for some family members to visit where their older relatives live, so they prefer to stay away. However, Moore's quality of spiritual attention belongs to their late life stage, whether or not dementia is present, and there is much that can be achieved to strengthen people with dementia through spontaneity and creativity (Casson, 1994).

A colleague in mental health care once said that client reha-bilitation 'has Harry Potter's cloak of invisibility thrown over it' (Rowling, 1997, cited by Still, 2009, personal communication); the same could be said of some facilities for the elderly. Lev-Aladgem, dramatherapist, writes of an Israeli care home where nearby sub-urban residents 'ignored it as if the place and its elderly inhabit-ants were completely invisible' (Lev-Aladgem, 1999). It is the very invisibility of older people and their spiritual, physical, mental and emotional needs that this book is attempting to address.

In Australia there could still be more funding for people with dementia, despite increases in past years. Funding is, higher than counterpart organizations in the UK, similar to Canada and much lower than the USA. Dementia funding in comparison to other OECD countries has recently been low to average (Access Economics report, prepared for Alzheimer's Australia, 2003), however government funding to such institutions as the Centre for Research on Ageing at Curtin University in Perth, Western Australia may have served to alter these statistics. Australia still needs to improve in comparison with the USA, where the total percentage of GDP spent on research is .025 as compared with .0015 in Australia (Low et al., 2008).

This chapter discusses the connection between dramatherapy and creativity and offers a definition of dramatherapy for people with dementia. It establishes that the arts in general, and creative arts therapy in particular, are able to offer healing for older people. It addresses the ways in which creative arts can help to heal deficits in the health of elderly people. Using examples from practice, guidance is given about how dramatherapy can be used and assessed for people with low- and high-dependency dementia. Finally, suggestions are given for future development of dramatherapy in training, research and implementation.

Creativity as a support to successful ageing

The healing properties of the arts were referred to by the ancients in many societies. In contemporary culture, especially within the twentieth and twenty-first centuries, there has been more consciousness that creative activity can contribute to people's health and well-being. Creative arts therapies emerged in Britain and the United States in the aftermath of Second World War, and art and music were seen to play a significant role in helping injured and traumatized veterans come to terms with the horrors of war (ABC Television Compass Programme, 2003). Drama joined these arts within hospitals, and practitioners began to discover the healing powers of creativity in group work (Jennings, 1975). The use of creative arts in occupational therapy has been highlighted (Miller & Fox, 1988) as well as the promotion of health through creativity

(Denshire, 2005) and creativity research in the ageing process recommends innovative ways to assist elderly people (Basting, 2009). Miller and Fox (1988) compare the maintenance of creativity in our lives as 'like having one foot in the valley and one in the mountains' – an ability to tolerate paradoxes and create order out of chaos – so important in dementia work (Miller & Fox, 1988). Among the arts therapies, whose evidence base for efficacy is ever becoming stronger, dramatherapy is emerging as a well-documented healing form of creativity and self-expression for dementia, an area where the creation of order from chaos can be so challenging.

Defining dramatherapy

What do dramatherapists do? Dramatherapy intentionally uses theatre and drama techniques to encourage the client's creativity and expressive ability.

Dramatherapy helps the clients to tell their story, express their feelings, set goals, extend inner experience and 'With drama therapy, (elderly people) are given the opportunity to redefine themselves, to revisit or reclaim their old roles, and to audition new roles they may want to acquire' (NADT website, 2009). The kinds of aims looked for by the dramatherapist are categorized as follows by the British Association for Dramatherapists:

> Effect psychological, emotional and social changes give equal validity to body and mind within the dramatic context engage clients with stories, myths, playtexts, puppetry, masks and improvisation enable the client to explore difficult and painful life experiences through an indirect approach. (British Association of Dramatherapists website, 2009)

The use of drama and theatre as an intentional means of change to facilitate growth is the essence of Dorothy Langley's approach (Langley, 2006). She says the intention differentiates dramatherapy from other forms of dramatic activity. Staying within the area of intention, there is usually an understanding and trust built-up between therapist and client which may include a discussion of client-centred goals.

Dramatherapy with people with dementia

There is valuable quantitative as well as qualitative evidence for the efficacy of dramatherapy with people with dementia. Schmitt and Froelich (2007) in a review of studies of creative therapies found that two studies used control groups in relationship to dramatherapy. The first study (Lepp et al., 2003) found that people with dementia in the dramatherapy group showed improved abilities in communication and confidence compared with the control group. In the second study which examined the combined use of dramatherapy and dance movement therapy, Wilkinson et al. (1998) found that members of the dramatherapy group had better cognitive function, daily living skills and lower dependency than those not in the group. Although none of the differences were significant, the findings support that creative therapies may help people accept dementia and cope with it better.

The dramatherapist uses many strategies such as role play and improvisation, mime, puppetry, storytelling, play and symbolic objects. The question may be raised however: are these strategies of the drama teacher, or recreational therapist? To answer this question, Joanne Hensman (2005) in her exploration of some differences between drama and dramatherapy with older people refers to the reintegration process. The dramatherapist has a range of strategies that may repeat this process in different ways. She gives, for example, Sue Jennings' 'Embodiment, Projection, Role' method. Here, the activities of embodying an emotion or feeling, projecting it onto an object or taking on a role follow the human developmental process of the young child (see Appendix 3.1). Because of this process, awareness of the sequencing of interventions is helpful, and this will be discussed later in the chapter. Meanwhile, the following techniques to assist people who have dementia are examined in greater detail.

Puppets and symbolic objects

There is a good case for using plenty of concrete material with this population. Using simple glove-puppets allows 'the silent and safer enactment of the clients' stories through the gradual revealing of the secret or the unspeakable' (Rowan,1966/7). It is not always necessary to work with sound, and silences and gesture can be just as powerful. Lev-Aladgem works with objects and describes how one older person used her beautifully carved walking stick as an object of focus. Her work emphasizes play with objects.

My own experience in mental health, for example with adolescents and people with addiction, as well as work with people with dementia is that, to begin with, the safe distance from the clients' potential issues is a contained and creative way to play. The dramatic projection is often the process by which clients recognize aspects of themselves or their experience in dramatic materials, thereby externalizing inner conflicts (Jones, 2007). In reminiscence therapy, it will promote life review (Langley, 2006). Clothes, pictures, objects and cards can assist with a smooth transition into play, story making and improvisation.

Play

Play is an important part of the range of techniques, and for people with dementia for whom confusion, withdrawal and depression is a way of life, play can be a pleasurable way of engaging. Kitwood (1990) recommends that a good care environment enables abilities to play (usually poorly developed in adults) to grow. Knocker (2001) is an experienced dementia care specialist and dramatherapist. She explores the connections between theoretical concepts and tools of dramatherapy, developmental psychology and current discussion on dementia care, establishing play as an efficacious activity for these clients.

Knocker disposes straightaway of the potential objection that the activity may be associated with the destructive infantalization of older people, quoted by Kitwood as a 'malignant social psychology' (Kitwood, 1990). She refers to her own training of care staff within dementia care and encourages exaggerated gestures and facial expressions, colourful clothing and what she calls 'talkative' eyes to engage interest and convey a mood with people with dementia with whom they are working.

Casson (1994) believes the therapist's responsibility is to enter into the client's chaos. He describes how he listens to the person with dementia with an ear to symbolic and affective content, hypothesizing that there might be emotional states the person is struggling to express that he could validate. He describes how he used this strategy with Laura, a potentially violent client, listening with his heart for feeling, rhythm and symbolism. She appeared to benefit from this validation and playful acceptance of her communication. After their interchange, he describes a playful dramatic situation where she chose a toy boat from a collection of playthings, and used it as a shoe, whereupon he became the shoe shop attendant, massaging her foot. He describes the interaction as one where she moved from hostile isolation to empathic contact with him, where her need for warmth and compassion was met.

Storytelling

Storytelling is extremely powerful for people with dementia; stories are the stuff of our shared humanity. When they and their mysterious atmospheres, movements and characters are missing for people of any age, there is a sense that people are being 'written on from the outside' in the insensitive and jangling language of the lower orders of media and technology (Keen, 1990).

Gersie (1997), who has spent many years studying therapeutic story making and the power of story, working with many populations to integrate the meaning of their lives – painful though this may be – tells of her work in a residential home for older people.

She captures the dichotomy that aged care workers often face between apparent compliance with the family and care home and the elderly people's very real interest in their own life stage.

> During story making I place great emphasis on the interactional and interpersonal here and now meanings of group members' overt behaviour and on their conscious wishes and expectations…They understood their task to be: how not to be a nuisance and how to die gracefully. However, in spite of their unwell bodies and sullen surface behaviour, these were also lusty, passionate, curious people

who wanted to surmount these unexamined confines of what old age was supposed to be about. (Gersie, 1997, p. 69)

Stories provide individuals with the means for the healing process. Role identification with the protagonist or others can help to recover lost or forgotten parts of the self. As long as a story 'holds together', many details can be left unexplored, and it can offer the chance of an alternative world (Grainger, 1990). It gives the participants the opportunity to understand aspects of their own biography through role identification with the characters. Certain fairytales can even be told which would bring a healing response in a particular organ of the body (Mellon & Ramsden, 2008).

A group of professionals in Sweden explored the healing potential of storytelling in people with dementia (Holm et al., 2004). The project was part of a larger undertaking, designed for people with dementia and their carers. Six strategically selected patients, with moderate or severe dementia, met for one and a half hours, once a week for two months. During this time, stories were exchanged between the participants that corresponded to the last stage of development in human beings (Erikson, 1982) which related to the acceptance of past life events. The study found that storytelling triggered many emotional responses and associative conversations. Storytelling as a tool was found to

- awaken memories,
- activate involvement and curiosity,
- invite participants to take part in existential conversations,
- help people to talk about difficult subjects.

The study acknowledged that the concept of co-working in this way needs further development and research on the effect storytelling has on the well-being and quality of life of people with dementia. Importantly, story telling for the people with dementia was a carer-initiated project, showing they saw potential for this work in the everyday care of patients.

There are other ways besides that of Erikson to look at various stages of human development. O'Neil and O'Neil (1990) see 63 to 84 years as mirroring the middle years from 21 to

42 years. Thus, for the healthy older person the first seven years up to the age of 70 is a period of adventure, discovering the world of retirement; the next years to 77 can be a time of 'dying and becoming' and the third period to the age of 84 is a renewal and resurgence of creative forces. These stages can also be borne in mind for the person with dementia, rather than offering life stages that are dominated by negative symptoms and weaknesses which often characterize some medicalized interventions. In the arts, familiarity and old illusions play pivotal roles. However, so do early life experiences, often the last memories to be lost in dementia because they are not subject to short-term or middle-term memory loss (Weisberg & Wilder, 2001).

Story making is an important intervention to bring the memories to consciousness and work with them.

Improvisation

My first experience of improvisation and dementia came as a young mother in her early 30s, working night shifts, with no knowledge of dramatherapy, as a nursing assistant in a home for elderly people. Mavis, who had dementia, would come downstairs in the middle of the night, informing her care worker that she could not return to bed, because her husband was still away and the roast dinner was ready. Up to the bedroom we would go, and I would ask Mavis to look out of the window for her husband Bob while she helped to 'prod the roast', and then got her to 'help set the table'. When everything was ready, and Mavis was sure she could hear Bob's footsteps on the stairs, she would get back into bed. Improvisation had solved the midnight wandering.

Improvisation may well follow on from storytelling – sometimes in unsuspected ways.

After some reflection on an improvisation on a story told about a generous and persistent old woman who went on a long, circuitous journey to search for apples to make an apple cake, a group member said: 'I need to be more patient.' This was especially significant as there was a participant present whom she had often criticized and her criticisms of that person ceased thereafter.

Johnson (1986) uses improvisation in a developmental manner, again using Erikson's model, to create meaning. His goal for sessions is to establish healthy interpersonal relationships among group members. In a case study, using a dramatherapy session with six people in a nursing home who are oriented with moderate cognitive impairment, he illustrates the pivotal role of the dramatherapist in creating personal (and group) significance.

The therapist may, at any time, enter into the role play by picking up on a group member's comment and transforming it into a new scene. In order to do this, the therapist must identify any developing image that seems to express a group theme. For example, when an action makes a distinction between good and bad children (perhaps connected with the patient's concern about their own children's infrequent visits), he takes an opportunity when various participants 'see' a skyscape:

> Therapist: OK, let's take all that good up there, the sky, the white cloud, and the rainbow...and bring it down, all together, bring it down and into ourselves (indicates by bringing arms down onto chest. Group follows in unison). (Johnson, 1986, p. 26)

In a less instantaneous example of the method of theme recognition using mixed media, Chin (1996) brings a small 'grief table' – a box with flowers and photograph – into the room after a member of the dramatherapy group has died. The installation is unacknowledged during the session. However, the following week when the box is there again to mark the end of winter with a butterfly inside and a sprouting bulb on top, a member with early late-stage Alzheimer's disease gets up, walks to the box and starts talking and weeping over friends who have recently died.

Each of these examples illustrates the need for concretizing feelings and 'going with' the theme of a dramatherapy group in a person-centred manner. In other words, humanity is being maintained in the face of diminishing cognitive powers and the potential for depression. The therapy takes the theme from the participants' verbal and non-verbal clues, and the facilitator works empathically from the viewpoint of the person. This method of working leads one to some practical suggestions to set up and structure a dramatherapy group of individuals with dementia.

Forming a dramatherapy group

It is helpful to consider the following principles when forming a dramatherapy group with people with dementia.

1. The therapist works with small group only – six or seven people to start with.
2. Assistance will be needed, not only for the comfort and mobility of people with low-dependency needs but also to observe for assessment purposes.
3. It is helpful to remember the care home's aims, as well as the therapist's and the clients'.
4. Even when people are unable to express themselves verbally, it is important to talk to other care workers and look at their care plans, so that an estimate of their aims can be made.
5. As Langley (1987) notes, a group of people with dementia and low-dependency needs may differ from those with high-dependency needs in their orientation in space, ability to take themselves to the toilet and so on. With varying levels of dementia among people in the group it is as well to have care workers to assist. Not only is this necessary to help people if they are confused or find it difficult to move around, but also for observation and assessment purposes. Even for those with low-dependency needs, helpers can assist with resources, repeating instructions and when needed, enhancing the general enthusiasm level.
6. Instructions should be clear about the time and the location of the group. It helps if the group can be designated as 'after morning tea' or 'before lunch', rather than ten or eleven o'clock.
7. It is also vital to have a room which is always used for the group, so that members are given every opportunity to remember the room in which the session is held at the same time each week, or twice weekly.
8. Most people with dementia usually understand clearly that this is 'therapy'. Whether or not this is the case, containment

is essential and a therapeutic contract: for example, no one interrupts, and time boundaries are kept.

9. Arrangements must be made to have the therapist's work supervised afterwards, ideally by an arts therapist or by a person with training and skills in working with groups. Supervision is an essential element in this work, for gaining insights and support and reviewing difficulties.

Assessment, goals and evaluation

It is important to know before commencing the dramatherapy how the group will be assessed. The aims for assessment of persons with dementia with low dependency may include

*   **physical exercise:** bodily movement involving physical flexibility;
*   **cognition:** memory orientation to present reality, with games and exercises around here and now routines, times and seasons;
*   **social orientation and life roles:** getting to know the self, other group members in a new way;
*   **self-expression and creativity:** personal reminiscence and cultural experiences;
*   **personal meaning and spirituality:** freedom and the meaning of life and death.

For people with higher-dependency needs these aims are also valid, although they may have to be assessed differently with simpler instructions, games, exercises and more concrete material, noticing more practical details such as the way people care for their appearance.

An assessment such as the Creative-Expressive Abilities Assessment is extremely useful in the arts therapies, and I have had a degree of success in reporting to the facility in a way that signposts future work, from using this tool (Gottlieb-Tanaka et al., 2008). It covers the areas of memory, attention, language, psychosocial, reasoning, emotion and culture/spirituality. Thus, valuable information about participants can be passed on to care staff. Evaluation forms can also be distributed to staff members, requesting information about the mood of participants afterwards, their comments and any effect on their well-being. This enables them to appreciate that achievements made later outside the group can have their origins inside it.

Beginning a dramatherapy group

Crimmens (1998) advises offering choice from the outset, bearing in mind our own thoughts and feelings as we go, giving people enough time and respecting the individual. She recommends adapting the format rather than expecting people to adapt to it. She points out that if people do not understand what is on offer, but feel they can trust the person who is offering it, they will probably want to go with the therapist.

There is much evidence that safety is of paramount importance early on in a group (Gersie, 1997; Stock Whitaker, 1992). A contract of some kind, containing information mentioned in the section on group formation, is valuable and sometimes, contrary to advice offered by care staff, is understood by most participants even though not verbally acknowledged. Picture cards can be used to demonstrate confidentiality, looking after the self and time boundaries. By making a confidentiality agreement where participants are included in the process, the therapist immediately shows respect for the integrity of the group and its members (Douglas, 1991; Stock Whitaker, 1992). Another aspect of safety is to leave time at the end of the group for proper reflection, so that any uncomfortable memories or feelings that have been stirred can be discussed (Andersen-Warren, 1996). Resources are important, and a room large enough for those who can move around. Andersen-Warren also has excellent advice on simplifying resources – for example, costumes can be representational – one unrestricting item of clothing can be used for role play, such as an apron or a waistcoat. I personally have found that varied colours and sizes of clothes are easy to use and can be draped over a person in a wheelchair. Choice of colour is very important for people who are selecting roles. The duration of a group should be between half an hour and one and a half hours, depending on the client group and concentration skills.

After contract information and introductions (remember that participants may not know each others' names, even if living in the same institution), name games with a soft ball given or thrown simultaneously with the name are helpful. Getting-to-know-you exercises can be well received, such as passing around a scarf and asking members to use it in whatever style they would like, then passing it on. The next person then mirrors their use of the scarf, and so on. Some participants may not be able to move, and will have to stay sitting for these activities. Movement encourages physical activity, even if in the chair, and this can include moving in tune with various types of weather, colour or music. From there, it is an easy step, perhaps in the next session, to move in tune with feelings, embodying these. After this, projection can be used and an object passed around for comment, such as 'this key reminds me of...', and as people become more comfortable with one another, a handshake, or a gesture could be given (see Appendix 3.1 for sequence rationale).

Already there will be a theme arising – it is helpful to notice what these kinds of activities remind people about. In the next session, concrete objects may be used, preferably an assortment. Targeted reminiscence objects from earlier life can come later, and role play based on these later still. There is evidence that objects or puppets give participants more emotional distance at first, before they identify their own emotions (Landy, 1983). If people with dementia are to gradually build-up trust in each other and the therapist, it is advisable to move slowly at first until they are comfortable with less distance from the material.

From the first day onwards there should be some kind of ritual ending for the session. This could be a song, a verse, a gesture – the group may find a way of providing this if the therapist does not. These people are living the last years of their lives, and endings are important; marking them will help with their grief process, as noted with the 'funeral table' example (Chin, 1996). A period of reflection, as shown in previous examples, can connect imaginary scenes with participants' lives and is existentially important.

Conclusion

By means of a stepwise, targeted building of sensory and imaginative experiences, people with dementia can be enabled to feel validated and to explore their mental, social, cultural and spiritual selves through the creativity engendered in a dramatherapy group. The careful setting up of a group, described above, which over time engenders trust and social engagement, allowing a shared focus through creativity, is greatly needed in dementia care.

More research is required in all the creative arts therapies, using care workers as in the storytelling example (Holm et al., 2004) with the addition of training as creative therapists, so that they can become integrated into the lives of institutions. Adequate funding needs to follow the growing evidence base of research in the area. In dramatherapy, control groups should be established similar to those mentioned earlier (Schmitt & Froelich, 2007) and where possible larger numbers of participants be monitored.

A great deal of work still has to be done in order that institutions and funding bodies take seriously the idea of arts therapies and the support they offer to people with dementia. So that our growing numbers of people with dementia become more visible, provision needs to be made for a regular time and space for clinically supervised groups. The maintenance of creativity in our institutions, as well as our homes for the elderly is essential, so that the dramatherapist does not walk into a barren ground, but a fertile one, in order to set up a group.

Professional development in creative therapies is another method of organizing this, so that staff experienced with this client group can train to be creative arts therapists. Funding is also needed for short courses as well as for professional training. Professional associations in USA, UK and Australia list short course information on their websites which can assist aspiring therapists (National Association for Drama Therapy (NADT), British Association of Dramatherapists (BADth), Australian & New Zealand Art Therapy Association (ANZATA) and Australian Creative Arts Therapy Association (ACATA)). It must be remembered, however, that a short course does not qualify staff as dramatherapists, and clinical supervision is necessary from a qualified person for the safety of all concerned. It is essential for the therapist to be aware of speaking and listening interactions with clients, and to reflect on the process. Communication requires self-awareness as well as skills (Kuhn & Verity, 2008).

Any of the techniques that have been elucidated here can be emphasized, depending on the sequence of sessions, the nature of the group and the skills of the creative therapist. The telling and retelling of stories strengthens the memory, biographical work and use of concrete material increases focus and stimulates personal memories, while improvisation allows a journey of imagination which can lead into areas of spiritual and existential questions.

The choice of a special group room and clear time boundaries will increase safety and prevent falls. Aims, including the institution's, as well as assessment methodology, are crucially decided upon before sessions start. Supervision arrangements need to be made, together with identifying management and care assistant(s). Staff and family members need to be consulted, to avoid misunderstandings. Elderly people should be asked (invited) in a way they are unlikely to refuse (Kuhn & Verity, 2008) to join the group. Levels of dependency need consideration – also life stage and personal history – so that the therapist can start 'where people are'.

Sessions begin with a contract, introductions and name games which are fun and creative. Colourful cloths, objects, hats, dressups and puppets, particularly those which invite reminiscence, should be provided. Games can be invented or accessed from a large range of available books listing drama warm-ups, making sure these are not too complex for the group. Work in early sessions can include objects, using music and song, graduating to stories inspired by these and working towards improvisation. Endings need special attention, as they concern the existential and spiritual needs of the participants.

The containment of therapeutic understanding and time-and-place-boundaries can serve as a warm enfolding of these elderly people. Life stage strengths, such as the intensification of memories, a sense of the presence of loved ones who have died and questions about their own mortality can be responded to creatively. As the population ages, and more of us fall prey to dementia, it is ever more important to bring life and creativity to these people, and to see them as treasured elders of our community.

Appendix 3.1   Embodiment, Projection and Role (EPR): a diagnostic tool

Embodiment – Projection – Role, or EPR, as it has become known, is a developmental tool by which we can work in a safe and structured way, in order to introduce people of any age to experiential dramatherapy work (Jennings, 1999). These are early markers of life stages:

Embodiment

In the young child, we can observe how her earliest experiences are mainly expressed physically, through bodily stimulus and senses. The infant moves and plays along with the world physically, in order to experience the world. This helps her to develop identity later on.

Projection

Here, the child relates more to the external world, beyond the body. There is a focus on toys and objects that belong to the outside world. During this stage, children explore their own relationships to objects, and stories can be dramatized through toys or dolls. Children even speak through their teddy or favourite doll: 'Teddy wants a drink.'

Role

Dramatic play becomes a new way of playing, and the child starts to distinguish between mundane reality and dramatic reality. Imitation is strong, and the role modelling that comes from parents and caregivers is played out.

Significance for dramatherapy with people who have dementia

Even though these three stages belong to early development in the human being, they can be a useful guide for therapists when working with adults of any age, including those with dementia. They have particular relevance in planning and structuring a dramatherapy session for elderly people. In other words, as a general rule embodiment exercises should come first, followed by use of objects and puppets and then role play and improvisation.

References

ABC Television Programme (17/8/2003). www.abc.net.au/compass (accessed 10 August 2009).

Access Economics prepared for Alzheimer's Australia (2003). *The Dementia Epidemic: Economic Impact & Positive Solutions for Australia.* www.alzheimers.org.au/upload/EpidemicFull ReportMarch2003.pdf (accessed 9 August 2009).

Andersen-Warren, M. (1996). *Creative Groupwork with Elderly People: Drama.* Milton Keynes: Speechmark Publishing Ltd.

Australia and New Zealand Arts Therapy Association (ANZATA). www.anzata.org (accessed 27 March 2010).

Australian Creative Arts Therapy Association (ACATA). www.acata. org.au (accessed 10 January 2011).

Australian Dementia Research: Current Status, Future Directions? A Report for Alzheimer's Australia. Paper 16. June 2008. www. alzheimers.org.au/upload/DementiaResearchJune08.pdf (accessed 6 August 2009).

Basting, A. (2009). *Forget Memory: Creating Better Lives for People with Dementia.* Baltimore: John Hopkin University Press.

Breines, E. B. (1995). *Occupational Therapy Activities from Clay to Computers.* Philadelphia: F.A. Davis.

British Association of Dramatherapists website (BADth). www. badth.org.uk (accessed 26 March 2010). (Note: *Dramatherapy* is the journal of this organization, and information can be accessed by emailing enquiries@badth.org.uk)

Casson, J. (1994). Flying towards Neverland. *Dramatherapy*, 16(2 & 3), 2–7.

Chin, C. (1996). Sounding board. Reconstructing the self with drama and creative arts therapies. *American Journal of Alzheimer's Disease*, 11(1), 36–42.

Crimmens, P. (1998). *Storymaking and Creative Groupwork with Older People.* London: Jessica Kingsley Publishers (pp. 28–29).

Denshire, S. (2005). Integrating the Firelight of Creativity: An Evolving Practice of Creativity-based Groupwork for Health and Well-being. In T. Schmid (ed.), *Promoting Health through Creativity* (pp. 148–166). London and Philadelphia: Whurr Publishers.

Douglas, T. (1991). *Common Groupwork Problems.* London: Tavistock Routledge (p. 118).

Erikson, E. (1982). *The Life Cycle Completed. A Review.* New York: Norton.

Gersie, A. (1997). *Reflections on Therapeutic Storymaking.* London: Jessica Kingsley Publishers (pp. 23, 69).

Gottlieb-Tanaka, D., Lee, H. & Graf, P. (2008). *Creative-Expressive Abilities Assessment: User Guide.* Canada: ArtScience Press.

Grainger, R. (1990). *Drama and Healing.* London: Jessica Kingsley Publishers (pp. 11–12).

Hensman, J. (2005). Some differences between drama and dramatherapy working with old people. *Dramatherapy,* 27(2), 18–22.

Holm, A., Lepp, M. & Ringsberg, K. (2004). Dementia: involving patients in storytelling – a caring intervention. A pilot study. *Journal of Clinical Nursing,* 14, 256–263.

Jennings, S. (ed.) (1975). *Creative Therapy.* London: Pitman.

Jennings, S. (1999). *Introduction to Developmental Play Therapy.* London and Philadelphia: Jessica Kingsley Publishers (pp. 51–53).

Johnson, D. (1986). The developmental method in drama therapy: group treatment with the elderly. *The Arts in Psychotherapy,* 13, 17–33.

Jones, P. (2007). *Drama as Therapy* (2nd Ed.). London: Routledge (p. 140).

Keen, S. (1990).*The Power of Stories Workshop.* Boulder, CO: Sounds True Recordings.

Kitwood, T. (1990). The dialectics of dementia: with particular reference to Alzheimer's disease. *Ageing and Society,* 10, 177–196.

Kitwood, T. (1997). *Dementia Reconsidered.* Buckingham: Open University Press.

Knocker, S. (2001). A meeting of worlds: play and metaphor in dementia care and dramatherapy. *Dramatherapy,* 23(2), 4–9.

Kuhn, D. & Verity, J. (2008). *The Art of Dementia Care.* New York: Thomson (pp. 41–45).

Landy, R. (1983).The use of distancing in dramatherapy. *The Arts in Psychotherapy,* 10,175–185.

Langley, D. (1987). Dramatherapy with Elderly People. In S. Jennings (ed.), *Dramatherapy Theory and Practice for Teachers and Clinicians* (p. 234). London: Croom Helm Publications.

Langley, D. (2006). *An Introduction to Dramatherapy.* Thousand Oaks, CA: Sage Publications, 1–2.

Langley, D. (2009). *An Introduction to Dramatherapy.* Thousand Oaks, CA: Sage Publications.

Lepp, M., Ringsberg, K. & Holm, A. (2003). Dementia – involving patients and their caregivers in a drama programme: the caregivers' experiences. *Journal of Clinical Nursing,* 12, 873–881.

Lev-Aladgem, S. (1999). Dramatic play amongst the aged. *Dramatherapy.* 21(3), 3–10.

Low, L- F., Gomes, L. & Brodaty, H. (2008). Australian Dementia Research: Current Status Future Directions. Report for Alzheimer's Australia. Paper 16, 21. http://www.alzheimers. org.au/upload/DementiaResearchJune08.pdf (accessed 7 March 2009)

Melbourne Institute for Experiential & Creative Arts Therapy (MIECAT). www.miecat.org.au (accessed 26 March 2010).

Mellon, N. & Ramsden, A. (2008). *Body Eloquence.* Fulton, CA: Energy Psychology Press.

Miller, V. & Fox, J. (1988). Creativity: The Forgotten Link in Occupational Therapy or One Foot in the Valley and One in the Mountains. Paper presented at the Australian Association of Occupational Therapists, 15th Federal Conference National Perspectives, Sydney, N.S.W.

National Association for Dramatherapy (NADT) United States of America. http://www.nadt.org (accessed 26 March 2010).

O'Neil, G. & O'Neil, G. (1990). *The Human Life.* New York: Mercury Press.

Rowan, C. (1966/7). Silence. *Dramatherapy,* 18(3), 12–14.

Rowling, J. K. (1997). *Harry Potter and the Philosopher's Stone.* London: Bloomsbury.

Schmitt, B. & Froelich, L. (2007). Creative therapy options for patients with dementia – a systematic review. *Fortschritte der Neurologie – Psychiatrie,* 75, 699–707. (German language only).

Stock Whitaker, D. (1992).*Using Groups to Help People.* London: Routledge (pp. 245–274).

Weisberg, N. & Wilder, R. (2001). *Expressive Arts with Elders.* London: Jessica Kingsley Publishers (p. 11).

Wilkinson, N., Srikumar, S., Shaw, K. & Orrell, M. (1998). Drama and movement therapy in dementia: a pilot study. *The Arts in Psychotherapy,* 2(3), 195–201.

4 Dance movement psychotherapy in dementia care

Richard Coaten

The aim of this chapter is to inspire readers to consider the nature and importance of arts-based practices that are embodied and that may help us to better understand the struggle that the person with dementia may have in order to communicate. This chapter is about providing new ways to support those processes of communication for people living with dementia, for their carers and professional care-staff, in homes, care homes, day centres and hospital wards. I present some of the ideas and embodied practices that have preoccupied me these past years, specifically in relation to the practice of Dance Movement Psychotherapy (DMP), and important ways in which its essence can be discussed, better understood and disseminated in books such as this.

DMP takes place in and through a living, breathing, moving body in the present moment, which means that to express this lived reality in *words* is to risk losing its essence, or missing the point in translation. It also risks losing the reader completely or boring them with jargon and technique. This chapter clearly communicates the essence of what using embodied practices mean, in spite of limitations found in translation and without being dogmatic; in order to inspire, to reach more people prepared to journey and explore for themselves what is at times both ordinary and also extraordinary about this work.

The chapter is not meant as a 'how-to' reference text as that is duplicating what I, and others, have attempted in other publications (Coaten, 2001; Coaten & Warren, 2008; Crichton, 1997; Garnet, 1982; Hill, 2001; Palo-Bengtsson, 1998; Perrin 1998; Meekums, 2002; Shustik & Thompson, 2001). It is meant to link to other work of a similar type, to support a well-argued case for the use of DMP in this field, giving short examples and to inspire the reader to explore and develop their own professional practise and their own creativity in using movement, dance and embodied practices.

In my doctoral thesis I carefully investigated what I understand by embodied practices and their significance, in relation to people living with dementia and those who care for them (Coaten, 2009), and I would therefore refer readers, who are interested in further study in this area, to this more detailed text. In this chapter I only sketch out what I mean by them as I intend to go further covering new ground for me, and hopefully others too. This attention towards and interest in 'embodied practices' are at the heart of being better able to reach the person through the body rather than through cognition and the intellect, where that is compromised and has to date been a neglected area of study and research in the field.

As a registered Dance Movement Psychotherapist I must state as a caveat that my own interest and involvement, in addition to my clinical practise, is to train and support care-staff and anyone else interested in the provision and development of embodied practices; it is not to turn them into dancers and/ or qualified and registered Dance Movement Psychotherapists. There are UK based Universities such as University of Derby, Roehampton University (London), and Goldsmiths University of London, Queen Margaret University (Edinburgh) and 'Dance Voice, Dance Movement Therapy Centre' in Bristol, ably providing courses as well as Master's in DMP.

The importance of embodied practices

The word 'embody' means to have or to hold something within the body in any number of ways, for example, metaphorically, physically, psychologically, emotionally, spiritually; in effect to live that 'something' through relationship with and in one's body. This definition assumes two things: first that we have a body in which we exist in the world, and second that we have access to the world through the body in which we experience it. These two assumptions imply relationship between the life and experience of the body per se (embodiment) and the reality of the world in which that body exists (corporeality). So far so good; analysis of the history of science from the time of the Cartesian mind/body split in the eighteenth century, however, has not been kind to the idea of body-presence as both an objective and a subjective reality. Scientific study has sought to delineate a so-called scientific 'objectivity' via denial of the fact that it is the 'body', its sensory perceptions and subjective, holistic ways of making sense of these perceptions that are at the heart of scientifically based investigations in the first place. The following description by a renowned pioneer of bodywork goes to the heart of this intimate relationship at the heart of embodiment:

> I both have a body and I am a body, and this intimate relation puts my body in a closer juxtaposition with my immediate awareness than any other object that I can possibly contemplate. No piece of laboratory equipment could ever put me closer to a form and its process of formation than can my direct perception of my own body. (Juhan, 1987, p. 11)

In the 1960s, a famous French philosopher was able to describe, analyse and challenge this denial regarding the importance of the lived body within the 'Phenomenology of Perception' (Merleau-Ponty, 1962) in a new way, addressing head-on the duality of the Cartesian mind/body split, by arguing in effect that it was a delusion, or what Abram (1996) has called a 'mirage':

> The common notion of the experiencing self, or mind, as an immaterial phantom ultimately independent of the body can only be a mirage: Merleau-Ponty invites us to recognize at the heart of even our most abstract cogitations, the sensuous and sentient life of the body itself. (Abram, 1996, p. 45)

As the body is the medium that alone enables us to be in relationship with the world and for the world to be in relationship with us, as human beings, then without the body there would be no possibility of experiencing the world. This logically presupposes that the body in and of itself is the true subject of experience, what Merleau-Ponty (1962) was to call the 'le corps sujet' or the 'body-subject'. For the time, this was a radical discovery about the centrality of the body in the phenomenology of perception and it was not well received by the psychiatric establishment for whom the body, backed up by the weight of biomedical science, focused predominantly in reductionist ways on better understanding body 'parts' in isolation, rather than in integrated 'wholes'. The reality and importance of the lived body for a person living with dementia and those who care for them are only recently being described and thought of as being of increasing importance in the everyday practise of care (see below). For example, the recent work of Sheard and colleagues epitomizes a different and much more embodied and emotionally congruent perspective, '(t)he rehabilitation of function has received more attention than restoring people's sense of being and spirit. Physical repair has taken greater precedence than the concept of emotional healing' (Sheard, 2009, p. 1).

Contemporary researchers in the past six years in the field of dementia have referred to the body in the literature for dementia as the 'lived body' (Dekkers, 2004; Kontos, 2005; Phinney & Chesla, 2003). The lived body is the body that is immediately apparent to me as I live and experience it. All that I sense, feel, touch and taste for myself is experienced, expressed and mediated through this, my body. Merleau-Ponty also proposed the idea that the lived body possessed its own knowledge of the world, what he called a 'tacit knowledge', and that this knowledge functioned outside of our conscious control. This subtle and implicit form of bodily-knowing is not based on cognition or cognitive processes but is inherent in our having a body and being human, it is indeed the basis upon which all perception takes place and ultimately all the decisions, movements, behaviours and communications we subsequently make. In relation to my own movement and dance training and my subsequent movement-based experiences in relation to the lived body, I have attempted to describe, what I have experienced as a relational and inter-subjective kind of intelligence and sensitivity that is available to us here:

Working from the intelligence of the body is about a process, not an outcome, which creates a spontaneous flow of information that is very different from intellectual information...the voice of the body rises when the intellect moves over. It doesn't offer diagnosis, treatment or cure, but contributes to an enriched awareness and understanding about how dis-ease manifests in and through the body. Insights occur through the movement itself, or through reflection and discussion following movement, and these can contribute to a greater understanding of what might be going on within oneself. (Coaten, 2000, p. 114)

What began as a gradual understanding of the importance of embodied practices that I was seeing and experiencing for myself then evolved, via much study and clinical practise, into a means whereby I could better appreciate and understand the significance of embodied practices for the people with whom I was working. What struck me most profoundly however, in relation to people with cognitive and memory problems, was that the application of these practices meant that I now had more effective ways of developing my relationships with them and they with me. My study also found that these practices provided support for residual capacities, such as the ability to reminisce, the ability to move and dance and by way of these, contributing to the concept of 'personhood' (Kitwood & Bredin, 1992, p. 274). They also contributed to, 'improving mobility; affirming identity; supporting affective communication; increasing observed "well-being" and extending the range and quality of care relationships' (Coaten, 2009, p. ii). Going by way of the body and embodied practices also meant working with non-verbal, body-based, emotionally congruent communications, without depending on the need for intact cognitive and intellectual processing. This 'tacit knowledge' (Merleau-Ponty, 1962) or implicit form of body-knowing gave me new ways to better understand wants and needs. It meant being able to get under-the-skin of the purpose and content of communication, both verbal and non-verbal, often with less duress on either myself or the 'other', and doing so in ways that enabled me to build what I have called, 'Bridges of Understanding' (Coaten, 2009, p. 9) between that about which I knew and was able to make sense of, and that about which was yet-to-be-known. Interestingly, this process is mirrored in a recent paper that has referred to 'the principle of building islands of contact' (Müller-Hergl, 2009, p. 15) in which the author similarly found ways to make time for contact with people with dementia in care homes, undisturbed by 'an ocean of pressing demands and tasks to be completed. It helps to cultivate hope' (ibid.). Cultivating hope reduces feelings of hopelessness and helplessness, while at the same time reducing observed 'ill-being'. Complexity and richness of non-verbal communications often involving humour are also present, while acknowledging the challenge that Ward has set out that, '...(a)s the recipients of care, people with dementia are best placed to comment upon the need for change. The challenge ahead lies in finding the best possible route to supporting their struggle to be heard' (Ward et al., 2002, p. 36).

What are embodied practices?

If I and others are right in our assumptions which still need more testing and research, then all involved in care practices have available an important and embodied creative medium for achieving Ward et al.'s challenge in 'finding the best possible route to supporting their struggle to be heard' (ibid.). Movement, dance and embodied practices help us find those best possible individually tailored routes in supporting that struggle as has been so well described by Hill (2001, p. 1), 'In the dance it was possible still to see and make contact with the individual. Despite the doom and gloom attached to dementia and the real hardships of the disease, people retained an ability to surprise and to do things that we did not think them capable of.' Thus movement and dance contribute embodied pathways that mediate between the person and their experience of the world and their struggle to have their communications heard, understood and acted upon. As a result, care processes can be more effective. I need to stress here that the use of embodied practices are not confined to the work of the Dance Movement Psychotherapist (of whom there may always be few in number) as they also offer important opportunities for carers, professional care-staff, nurses and others to reconfigure their understanding and use of the lived body in care practices that are more embodied and therefore more relational.

I understand the use of embodied practices, as I have described them here, taking place in two principal areas that I will now discuss and give examples of. The first concerns the use of 'Embodied Practices involving Movement and Dance' and the second the use of 'Embodied Practices in Everyday Care'. With regard to the former I have chosen to focus on aspects of my own experience and practise relating specifically to care-staff training, as the details of embodied practices in relation to movement and dance have been covered by myself and others in earlier publications.

Embodied practices involving movement and dance

This area has as its principal focus the provision of group and one-to-one, movement and dance-based sessions on a regular basis that use embodied practices where often words are no longer necessary or are of less importance. The provision of these practices requires training for those seeking to embark on their use, and as a part of the process much can be gained by studying the work of those writers and clinicians, already referred to, who have documented their own approaches and recommendations in this regard. Better still is to be able to take part in an actual training programme that is specifically focused on gaining knowledge, skill and experience in this area that is of the embodied and experiential kind. This work is relatively new and evolving at this time in the UK, and unfortunately as I write there are no programmes running that I am aware of that are open to any interested individuals wherever based. Perhaps the reader can be the first to consider setting one up themselves in their own location based on the ideas presented here.

Detailed aspects of the provision of a typical training programme cannot be discussed at great length here; however pointers can be given as to the essential characteristics of a high-quality training programme, in order to generate interest in them. Participants can include care-staff, carers, nurses, support time recovery workers, physiotherapists, occupational therapists, community dance workers and dance artists among others. From my own practise and research the following are worth considering as key aspects of the syllabus of a training programme that may last about three months.

Provision of a day's training in Person-Centred Care (PCC)

The focus of this off-site day lays the foundations of embodied practices, rooting them in core values and principles that increase awareness and understanding of the importance of concepts such as Positive Person-Work (Kitwood, 1997, pp. 90–93) 'personhood' (Kitwood & Bredin, 1992, p. 274) and the more contemporary summation of PCC as provided by the 'VIPS' Framework (Brooker, 2007, p. 112). The day can include a variety of different approaches including showing films, carrying out experimental and group-based exercises and discussions around problem-solving and case studies. It is helpful to evaluate the day and also for participants to have a key goal committing them to making one significant change to their care practices as a result of the training.

Provision of off- and on-site training experiences

Following a one day training in PCC, which provides an excellent foundation for what is to come, further off- and on-site work enable exploration of the key themes, introducing participants in experiential ways to the importance of the lived experience of the moving body; to those pathways of perception and awareness that are the building blocks of our own identity and integrity and that help maintain our sense of self. It also allows participants to truly experience the power of movement and dance work for themselves, first during carefully planned and structured off-site training, where they cannot be disturbed and called away by their colleagues, followed by on-site implementation delivered by the trainer/trainers. The approach does require participants to have initially experienced and appreciated it by literally 'doing it', followed by the learning of specific skills, knowledge and ability in how to provide and pass on sessions on a group and individual basis. It is ideal, if following or alongside several off-site training days, on-site sessions take place facilitated by the trainer/trainers, with a gradual handover of session facilitation to the trained staff after a period of 5/6 weeks of implementation.

As 'movers' we remember that in working in and through the body, we work with all of a person's life experiences stored in skin, in muscle and in bone. Given the right triggers or stimulae these can and do return, re-membered as living symbols of the original event manifesting in the present moment. This means care staff/carers learning how to become more attuned to providing and also maintaining vital individual sensory, physical, psychological, emotional and spiritual resources that tap into residual capacity while supporting and maintaining 'personhood' (Kitwood & Bredin, 1992, p. 274). In my experience where people may have had careers as dancers or have loved to dance, the process described above can become even more significant and of profound importance to someone with a dementing condition as well as to their family.

Provision of a wide-ranging syllabus – movement and dance skills

A syllabus needs to include the skills and techniques of movement and dance-based practices, concerning successful group and one-to-one based implementation over the short, medium and long term. The crucial question, however, is how to enable and inspire trainees to become much more aware of their own creativity, their own interest in and feelings for movement and dance, and how these new skills and ideas might be successfully implemented in their own care settings? I readily accept and clearly state my position in any training on this subject, that whilst I can provide experiences that inspire and support the use of these practices, I am not teaching a 'model', rather an 'approach'. This 'approach' is not dogmatic; it is best learned in embodied and experiential ways and has many different elements to it. I am supporting trainees to read the runes, the hieroglyphics of dementia, doing so through embodied practices, through the language of metaphor and symbolism, through rhythmic movement, melody and music and through the use of particular techniques such as 'Mirroring' (Levy, 1992): I also use group and individual structures and a variety of different props including scarves, cloth, fans, large and small pieces of elastic aiming to support memory, communication and the maintenance of physical, psychological, emotional and social resources. By supporting individual capabilities and resources, people with dementia can thus be helped to remain living independently in their communities for as long as possible.

Participants can take away and use what is provided during a training programme; however, the reality of how that is transferred and used with people living with dementia is profoundly dependent on a number of factors. These include, for example, the quality of the relationships made between group members, the values propounded, the skills of the facilitator in presenting the material and the comfort and ease with which people are enabled to participate, to name a few of the variables. As in learning any new skill, beginning with confidence in the medium, the approach used, together with a sense of flow to the session may be lacking. It can help a great deal to have both off- and on-site training provision so participants are able to witness on-site how the work looks and feels in a group of people with whom they are already familiar. In this way the use of embodied practices involving movement and dance can be embedded in the practise of care.

Provision of a wide-ranging syllabus – forming and running groups

This aspect presupposes that the approach needs grounding in the realities of people using it being able to set-up, maintain and run groups on a short- or long-term basis if necessary. The title therefore is a simpler way of referring to skills in the leadership and management of groups taking place in venues of different kinds. These can range from lounges in care homes, to community halls and even to suitable outside spaces when the weather is warm enough and the space conducive to the group. Key to this aspect of the syllabus is for participants to be given some theory, knowledge and skills about how to run groups successfully and for this learning to take place initially off-site. Once the on-site work begins participants can observe how the training programme facilitator runs sessions with their own residents, and also how they respond to the unique challenges and on-site opportunities presented by the setting and the people. In Figure 4.1, I have found a helpful way of identifying the main theoretical aspects of the session and for it also to be used as a helpful diagnostic tool:

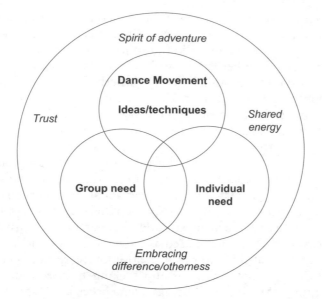

Figure 4.1   Theoretical aspects of forming and running groups

Here the three interlocking circles represent the three main aspects of a session, the Dance Movement ideas/techniques, the needs of the group and the needs of the individual. These take place within an outer circle or 'overall atmosphere' that visually expresses the idea of four essential characteristics. There needs to be present in the session a 'spirit of adventure', a 'shared energy', a sense of being able to trust each other (which builds over time) and most important perhaps, the ability to accept and even embrace aspects of 'difference/otherness' and ambiguity that are essential to working with groups of this type. The goal of the session as expressed visually and theoretically through the diagram is represented by the middle space where the three interlocking circles meet. If the session facilitator can effectively meet all these different needs then the session is likely to have been a memorable and effective one in achieving its goals. If, on the other hand, this is not the case, then by using the diagram diagnostically it is possible to make certain inferences. For example, whether or not the movement/dance ideas presented were appropriately chosen for the group at that time. Whether or not the group and/or individual needs were being effectively catered to. Whether or not the overall atmosphere was conducive to the work in hand. Other factors such as room temperature, room size, location, staff availability and whether or not the session is happening in private or taking place in the main lounge are also important. A session taking place surrounded by other residents in a main lounge for example, whose presence is not engaged by the group and its activities, is not conducive to it working out well. In this case the three interlocking circles in the diagram above may reflect an imbalance, as group and individual needs may not have been adequately met, coupled perhaps with the overall atmosphere reflecting a lack of trust also negatively influencing the desired outcome. Apart from the diagram above being used as a diagnostic tool, it can also be used to contribute to the evaluation of the session, perhaps within the context of the group seeking to raise individual and group observed 'well-being'. Dementia Care Mapping has also been used in research and evaluation of the use of movement and dance with results indicating significant increases in observed 'well-being' (Coaten, 2009; Crichton, 1997; Perrin, 1998).

Embodied practices in everyday care

This second aspect of embodied practices is new to me as I write this, is less clearly defined and has emerged in response to the question I recently asked myself. If I am clear about the use of embodied practices using movement and dance having witnessed their positive effects over many years, are they still relevant to people who don't want to take part in movement and dance work? I began to consider ways in which care practices might become more embodied without the use of dance, especially with people for whom that kind of activity would not have engaged them at other times in their lives. Trying to answer this question helped me to observe more acutely the embodied aspects of the care practices that I was seeing in my everyday work settings, which inevitably raised more questions. For example, how were my colleagues engaged on a daily basis with day-attenders involving movement and touch? Also how was I for that matter engaged with day-attenders outside of any formal DMP session? Were care-staff and day-attenders comfortable with the embodied practices that involved movement rather than dance, and if not how did they show it? What messages could be identified by someone who was walking around a lounge or entrance area looking confused, might they need help and could I offer a hand or simply my body-presence in that regard? Offering body-presence meant that one simply accompanies the 'other' while walking between places, or while sitting or just being together; perhaps resisting the need for small talk. What I realized was that this quality of walking or being together presented opportunities for developing attentiveness to how I was responding to the other person and they to me. It might be described as a 'tuning-in' to the other person rather as one attunes to the group and individual during a movement and dance-based session. In the example quoted here, there is a meeting that takes place with the possibility for creating what Dance Movement Psychotherapists describe as the therapeutic alliance based on essential qualities of trust, respect and that fundamental importance of what Kitwood has described as '... an I-Thou form of meeting' (Kitwood, 1997, p. 12). It means that in spite of biomedical thinking and training that seeks distance from the subjective and the inter-subjective in order to seek clarity, we must, if we seek to work in truly person-centred ways, learn how best to tune-in to what is and is not being said. Here the subjective and the inter-subjective become one where theoretically and practically clarity is established in and through relationship, through emotional intelligence and in ways so ably described by the recent work of Sheard (2009).

Psychologically there is a sense here of the person with dementia being well supported without the use of words, offering opportunities for expression of different personal qualities, such as self-worth, personal choice and autonomy, which as a process becomes of increasing significance as language deteriorates and word-finding and verbal expression become harder. Without the stress of word-finding the application of non-verbal techniques also supports a lessening of anxiety and tension and more attention to the ongoing process of how we understand ourselves. Here I reach a point where words seem inadequate to describe the flux and flow of our embodied communications, especially in relation to movement and touch, as it is a sensitive subject. Touch is of great importance to people compromised cognitively and struggling in so many ways to cope with the manifold losses involved. I have found the holding of a hand between my own, especially when a person may be upset or simply needing reassurance can communicate more effectively than many words. Reassurance and the reduction of observed 'ill-being' can be achieved effectively through emotionally congruent embodied practices, including the holding of a hand or hands and walking with someone with a greater attunement to the importance of embodied practices in the care-context as described above. I have referred to walking and hand-holding as two examples of what I mean, however almost all care practices involving bodily movement and action can be carried out with a greater attention paid to embodied awareness.

This section can only allude very briefly to the importance of embodied practices that are based on care-staff and others being more 'creatively alert' (Coaten, 2000, p. 110) to the importance of their own 'embodiedness' in the care situation, and how it may contribute much to developing more effective care practices.

Conclusion

In my opinion, for all those tasked with the care of people living with dementia at whatever age, or stage of the condition, there is an urgent need for a heightened embodied awareness using embodied practices that help the person find the best possible routes for communication, within a context of care being far more emotionally engaged. This call echoes that by Tom Kitwood back in 1997 when he so prophetically invoked us then, in his last publication, to assemble a new sentient humanity in and through the condition, kindling what he called 'our true interdependence' (Kitwood, 1997, p. 144) as human beings, and in the process helping reveal, 'an immeasurably richer conception of the human mind' (ibid.). The focus today must be to build on that prophetic call, still very relevant, that as care providers we open ourselves up to these different kinds of embodied practices, moving forward our understanding of the many different ways in which the lives of people with dementia can be enriched, in spite of all that diminishes. More research is needed to further investigate the results achieved so far in this field of DMP and dementia care, to disseminate findings and so contribute to furthering knowledge about the important practices described here within the context of Person-Centred Care.

Appendix 4.1 – An individual example

The following is a relaxing movement and dance-based activity for a carer and their loved one with dementia published in an arts-based recipe book for carers in the Calderdale area of West Yorkshire, England (Coaten, 2008). I am grateful for the organization's permission to reproduce it here. It is for doing at home rather than in a group or in public. 'Recipe Part 1' (ibid., p. 22) invites the carer to identify a comfortable place and a suitable time to start playing some relaxing music first; then to warm-up the hands of their loved one using hand cream or massage oil and to 'take this opportunity to "travel with", be a companion "for" the person wherever they go in their thoughts, ideas and feelings as you gently massage their hands' (ibid., p. 22). The second part is as follows:

'Recipe Part 2' – hand moving/dancing

1. Invite the person to see how their hands might like to move, now that they have been given some tender loving care.
2. Ask them if the nice music makes them want to gently move, stretch their fingers and/or hand(s).
3. You gently 'mirror', if you can, the person's movements, meaning that you join in with this hand moving/dancing experience. You may like to hold the hand or place your palm on theirs and see where this takes you both. Don't rush or hurry this, it may take some time for something to happen. It may take you off the chairs and into moving and/or dancing together – you can listen to the rhythm and tempo of the music and go with that – if it is relaxing you might even like to use a scarf (silk) and see where that takes you – you might find that you have a feather (peacock or pheasant or even ostrich) in the house and could explore its use as a prop with your person, (ibid., p. 23).

The most important aspect of this experiential work, as you try it out, is to remember to take pleasure in it all. If it can remain pleasurable, observed 'well-being' will have increased and 'ill-being' decreased. Together, you will have played and danced in embodied ways that truly offer hope in going by way of the body in dementia care, when words are not enough. I wish you well in your explorations in these growing and important 'embodied' practices.

References

Abram, D. (1996). *The Spell of the Sensuous*. New York: Vintage Books.

Brooker, D. (2007). *Person-Centred Dementia Care – Making Services Better.* London: Jessica Kingsley.

Coaten, R. (2000). Creating a Little Revolution – The Patient as Artist. In P. Greenland (ed.), *What Dancers Do That Other Health Workers Don't.* Leeds: Jabadao, 101–122.

Coaten, R. (2001). Exploring reminiscence through dance and movement. *Journal of Dementia Care,* 9(5), 19–22.

Coaten, R. (2008). Movement Matters. In Marsden, S. & Turner, J. (eds), *The Family Arts Recipe Book – A Recipe Book of Creative Ideas to Inspire* (pp. 22–23). Calderdale, UK: Verd de Gris.

Coaten, R. (2009). Doctoral thesis: *Building Bridges of Understanding: the use of embodied practices with older people with dementia and their care-staff as mediated by Dance Movement Psychotherapy.* Roehampton University, London, http://roehampton.openrepository.com/roehampton/handle/10142/90376

Coaten, R. & Warren B. (2008). Dance, Developing Self-Image and Self-Expression through Movement (3rd Ed.). In B. Warren (ed.), *Using the Creative Arts in Therapy and Healthcare – A Practical Introduction.* London: Routledge, 64–88.

Crichton, S. (1997). Moving is the language i use, communication is my goal. *Journal of Dementia Care,* 5(6), 16–17.

Dekkers, W. (2004). Autonomy and the Lived Body in Cases of Severe Dementia. In R. Purtilo & H. ten Have (eds). *Ethical Foundations of Palliative Care for Alzheimer Disease.* Baltimore: John Hopkins University Press, 115–130.

Garnet, E. D. (1982). *Movement Is Life – a Holistic Approach to Exercise for Older Adults.* Hightstown, NJ: Princeton Book Co.

Hill, H. (2001). *Invitation to the Dance: Dance for People with Dementia and Their Carers.* Dementia Services Development Centre, Stirling: University of Stirling.

Juhan, D. (1987). *Job's Body: A Handbook for Bodywork.* Barrytown, NY: Station Hill Press.

Kitwood, T. (1997). *Dementia Re-Considered the Person Comes First.* Buckingham: Open University.

Kitwood, T. & Bredin, K. (eds) (1992). Towards a theory of dementia care personhood and well-being. *Ageing and Society,* 12, 269–287.

Kontos, P. (2005). Embodied selfhood in Alzheimer's disease: rethinking person-centred care. *Dementia, International Journal of Social Research and Practice,* 4(4), 553–570.

Levy, F. (1992). *Dance/Movement Therapy: A Healing Art* (Revised edition). Reston, VA: American Alliance for Health, Physical Education & Dance.

Meekums, B. (2002). *Dance Movement Therapy, a Creative Psychotherapeutic Approach.* London: Sage.

Merleau-Ponty, M. (Translated by C. Smith) (1962). *The Phenomenology of Perception*. London: Routledge.

Müller-Hergl, C. (2009). Accept people as they are. *Journal of Dementia Care*, 17(3), 15.

Palo-Bengtsson, L. (1998). *Dancing as a Nursing Intervention in the Care of Persons with Dementia*. Stockholm, Sweden: Karolinska Institute.

Perrin, T. (1998). Lifted into a world of rhythm and melody. *Journal of Dementia Care* 6, 1, 22–24.

Phinney, A. & Chesla, C. (eds) (2003). The lived body in dementia. *Journal of Aging Studies*, 17, 283–299.

Sheard, D. (2009). *Nurturing Our Emotions at Work in Dementia Care*. London: Alzheimer's Society.

Shustik, L. & Thompson, T. (eds) (2001). Dance/Movement Therapy, Partners in Personhood. In A. Innes and K. Hatfield (eds), *Dance/Movement Therapy: Partners in Personhood* (Bradford Dementia Group Good Practice Guides). London and Philadelphia: Jessica Kingsley Publishers, 49–78.

Ward, R., Vass, A. A., Aggarwal, N., Garfield, C., Cybyk, B. & Minardi, H. (eds) (2002). Dementia, communication and care: 2. communication in context. *Journal of Dementia Care*, 10(1), Nov/Dec, 33–37.

5 Music therapy in dementia care

Kirstin Robertson-Gillam

Introduction

This chapter explores what music therapy is and how it can be applied therapeutically to raise the quality of life in people with dementia. It reports on music therapy research showing evidence of its efficacy in dementia care and offers ideas for carers and families to enhance their relationships and caring experiences.

Sacks's (2007) assertion that 'music of the right kind can serve to orient and anchor a patient when almost nothing else can' highlights how the uniqueness of music can impact a person with dementia. Music makes audible the essential personhood of individuals within the context of their own society and culture. It can be used for creating a deeper sense of coherence and resilience through which a person may grow and become healed from existing imbalances in their current health status.

Music therapy is the planned and applied use of music for therapeutic purposes and relationship-building. It is person-centred and involves deep spiritual and emotional connections between therapist and client. Music therapists are musicians who are trained both in music and in understanding human nature from biophysical, psychological and musical perspectives. The interactive nature of music involves both musical and verbal dialogue.

In all its forms, music has been found to be an effective communicative tool for people with dementia. The inability to convey thoughts and ideas are some of the first symptoms which challenge people with dementia. Music is a non-verbal art form, providing an avenue for spiritual, emotional and

cultural expression which can reflect the personhood of someone who lives with dementia. Music, especially singing, has
been found to stimulate the brain and energize the spirit
(Cohen, 2006), thereby increasing quality of life for people
who find themselves lost in a world of strangeness that typifies
the dementing process.

The following vignette illustrates these points:

Case study

Hubert (not his real name) was a retired school principal living with
dementia in hostel care. He had been a music teacher and thought
that his fellow residents were the children whom he had taught all
those years ago. When I gave him the role of conducting music therapy sing-alongs, he felt that he was back in his school room again. He
liked to look up the suggested song and read out the lyrics. The group
responded to Hubert each time and all joined in singing with great
pleasure and enjoyment. Many ideas and memories were retrieved
and expressed with these song themes. Each person in the group felt
validated. Hubert sang beautifully and felt satisfied and happy after
each group singing session.

A special moment occurred between us when Hubert began
to spontaneously play a rhythmic phrase on a tambourine which
I answered back to him on the piano. He repeated the phrase and
extended it, waiting for me to answer him once more. We continued
in this fashion, building and rebuilding our musical conversation. This
created a dynamic and creative interaction which helped to reduce
his late afternoon agitation. Over time, Hubert became more relaxed
and contented. He was able to express his personhood in the most
meaningful way through music. The positive feelings engendered by
this experience generalized into other areas of Hubert's life so that
he was able to relate more positively to others and this showed up as
a significant decrease in his levels of agitation.

'Music is what human beings are. It is the mirror of human
physical and emotional energy transformed into sound' (Schneck &
Berger, 2006, p. 28).

Historical aspects of music therapy

Music therapy began as a profession after the Second World
War when musicians were engaged to help soldiers suffering
from war trauma. Early anecdotal evidence pointed to the
effectiveness of music as an intervention to relieve depression

in people with dementia. Bright (1991) asserted that 'music brings a sense of individuality and a personal approach despite the decay of every other faculty' (p. 29). Other authors believe that singing could be regarded as a welcome release from the helplessness of being a patient, allowing thoughts to be communicated externally (Morgan & Tilluckdharry, 1982).

'To speak of music therapy is to speak of communication' (Benenzon, 1992, cited in Gaertner, 1999). Elderly people often find difficulty in communicating their needs. This can be due to biological trauma such as stroke or dementia, or by the simple problem of not being listened to because of their age.

Historically, music therapy in aged and dementia care was not widely documented until the late 1980s. Whereas in Great Britain, applied music therapy used live musical interactions with the therapist as in clinical improvisation (Odell-Miller, 1995), in the United States, live music was used as a teaching and learning tool focused on changing behaviours (Palmer, 1977; Schoenberger and Braswell, 1971). Early applications of music therapy in the United States were believed to be more focused on 'the patients fitting in with the therapist's music rather than vice versa' (Odell-Miller, 1995, p. 88).

Odell-Miller measured the cumulative effects of engagement during and after weekly music therapy sessions, using instrument and voice-building improvisations from the sounds and music expressed by group members. She found there were more sustained and higher levels of engagement during and after the music therapy sessions.

Early anecdotal evidence suggested that people with dementia may retain music function while language and social skills were diminished (Bright, 1972, 1991, p. 29). This assertion was later validated (Cohen, 2006; Crystal et al., 1989; Cuddy & Duffin, 2005; Miller et al., 2000; Sixsmith and Gibson, 2007).

Kenny believed that the musical experience of singing and making music provides 'an intimate link between sensation and consciousness; the space between Self and the World' (Kenny, 1989, p. 55). People with dementia live in a world that no longer makes sense to them. However, when singing and music-making occur, a sense of coherence can be experienced.

Case study

Dorita (not her real name), an animated elderly lady, attended my weekly music therapy reminiscence group set up as an afternoon tea party with musical instruments, pine cones, sea shells, spinning tops, small dolls, teddies and other objects.

Dorita had been a seamstress and was closely observing a New Zealand toy sheep. She voiced her concern that 'its eyes were hidden' and suggested that maybe it was short sighted! This generated much humour and animated discussions within the group.

The whole group became so energized that they eagerly reached for musical instruments and began playing and singing their favourite songs. Each group member demonstrated a sense of coherence, enjoyment and motivation. Their spirits soared and they each expressed their personhood in their own unique fashion. Sacks (2007) asserted that people with dementia never really lose their unique personality traits. This phenomenon was evident in these music therapy reminiscence groups.

Historically, Aldridge (1996, 2005) pointed out that music therapy articles about aged care focused mainly on group work (Christie, 1992; Olderog-Millard & Smith, 1989). Music therapy group activities were reported to increase socialization, communication, purposeful interactions with others as well as sensory and muscular stimulation and gross and fine motor skills (Segal, 1990). Some studies by Clair (1996; 2000) reported that participation in group music activities over a period of 15 months continued even though participants' cognitive, physical and social abilities decreased markedly.

Fitzgerald Cloutier (1993) compared reading to singing with an 81-year-old woman with dementia in order to analyse her attentiveness and wandering. Results showed that the singing sessions were more successful at keeping her seated and focused than the reading sessions. This research is instructive for carers who may be thinking of trying reading, playing music or singing favourite songs with a person who has dementia and may be exhibiting agitated behaviours.

More recent music therapy studies on dementia care

Hays and Minichiello (2005) used recorded classical music every evening in a dementia-specific facility to decrease the symptoms of agitation. Results indicated that music can contribute towards increasing self-esteem, enhancing feelings of competence and independence and lessening the experience of social isolation which is so evident in people with dementia. Delirium, as a result of infection, can also present as agitated and confused behaviour.

In the following case vignette, a daughter had felt distressed because her mother was confused and not recognizing her anymore. She learnt that symptoms of delirium will subside once the source of the infection has been treated.

Case study

A woman with dementia was suffering with a urinary tract infection and had become very confused. She wandered into the day room singing loudly. She sat down and vocalized in the most creative fashion. I responded with improvised vocalizations, thereby building up a musical conversation. She related to me with meaningful eye contact and began to have a conversation through song. She sang about the weather, clothes and other observations. At one stage, she sang a long note with me, sharing a moment of deep meaningful eye contact. We became linked and synchronized through the acoustic energies of our voices and emotional contact. She was able to hear and transform her utterances into meaningful communications because someone was there who listened and responded. 'Music forms and transforms human emotional and physical energies into acoustic energies that reflect and parallel in synchrony with the physiological system' (Schneck & Berger, 2006, p. 28).

This experience related to Brown's (2001) theory of 'musilanguage' in which 'music and language are seen as reciprocal specializations of a dual-natured referential emotive communicative precursor whereby music emphasizes sound as emotive meaning and language emphasizes sound as referential meaning' (p. 271). It seems possible that as a person becomes less able to communicate due to dementia, music can 'cut to the quick, requiring no semantic definition or explanation' (Schneck & Berger, 2006, p. 30).

Music therapy and brain plasticity

Miller et al. (2000) found that 'patients with left-sided temporal lobe dementia offer an unexpected window into the neurological mediation of visual and musical talents' (p. 1). It seems that damage to this part of the brain can unblock the potential for creative activity (Miller et al., 1998). This work validates earlier anecdotal evidence that music function as well as artistic function may remain, even in the face of increasing cognitive impairment (Bright, 1972, 1991; Clair, 1996).

Peretz et al.'s study (2004) found that nonmusicians were highly consistent in their ability to sing familiar songs. This phenomenon could be due to early childhood learning. They had precise memory for pitch and tempo. Other studies demonstrated that this precision was retained 'when measuring consistency across individuals in the sung recall of a popular song' (Levitin, 1994; Levitin & Cook, 1996, cited in Peretz et al., 2000, p. 3).

Peretz et al. (2004) also found that the tune and text of a song were 'heard and learnt together ... and the recognition of text and tune in song is mediated by distinct pathways' (p. 6). The 'singing route' in the brain would 'involve the store in which words were embedded in melodies' (p. 7). These studies support the use of well-known songs from earlier years to engage people with dementia. By singing the songs of earlier times, elderly people can learn to enjoy and trust the experience of music-making which can then lead on to spontaneous music-making or singing improvisation. In fact, with decreased inhibitions, people with dementia are enabled to express their personhood more effectively through spontaneous music-making.

Cabeza's (2002) study showed that the brains of older adults tended to be less lateralized than younger brains. Such bilateralized brain function appears to be a phenomenon of middle to later life where the brain is able to benefit from activities involving beauty and engrossing stimulation, integrating left and right brain involvement.

Cohen (2006) asserted that 'creative activities [such as improvisation, dancing or choir singing] challenge the older brain and that these types of activities and new experiences can induce the sprouting of new dendrites, thereby enhancing brain reserve' (p. 10).

Uddin et al. (2006) investigated the phenomenon of 'self-other discrimination' as being fundamental to social interaction through the neural systems that underlie this ability. Because people with dementia gradually lose the ability to recognize themselves or their family members and friends, this research offers a deeper understanding of our neural mechanisms and, in particular, what is called the 'mirror neuron system' which relates to how we learn by imitation. Music is unique in its ability to demonstrate and teach new skills through observation and imitation. As people with dementia progress through this creative process, they gain a sense of mastery and motivation. These positive emotions can lead to a boost in the immune system, thereby enhancing overall health (Kiccolt-Glaser et al., 2002).

Fukui and Toyoshima (2008) found that 'music listening and playing facilitates the neurogenesis, regeneration and repair of cerebral nerves by adjusting the secretion of steroid hormones, ultimately leading to cerebral plasticity'. Their study indicates that music is not only therapeutic but might be a necessary part of everyday life for a person with dementia. It seems that music could be seen as a medical intervention which promotes brain growth and awareness for all human beings.

Many studies have shown the positive effects of music on the social, psychological, physical and emotional states of the human system. These recent studies shed light on the dynamics of how music actually affects the brain as well as being a safe, cost-effective and potent therapeutic intervention which increases the quality of life for people with dementia and enhances relationships with their carers and their existing world.

Theories underpinning music therapy related to dementia care

Psychoanalytic theory

Winnicott (1971) was interested in the idea of the space between the inner and outer worlds as being a virtual world, a transitional space for play and creativity.

Winnicott felt that the task of the therapist was to provide a holding environment for the client in order for them to meet neglected ego needs and allow the true authentic self to emerge. Transitional objects including musical instruments, pine cones, sea shells, books and soft toys can act as intermediaries for exploring and working within the holding environment. Winnicott's ideas fit well with music therapy, especially clinical improvisation techniques and singing at individual and group levels. Making music is literally 'playing' in the most creative sense.

Case study

Mary (not her real name) had hearing loss as well as moderate dementia and regularly attended a weekly music therapy reminiscence group. During music-making, she surprised me with her complex rhythmic improvisations. She told me that she had been a music teacher and a long-term member of a church choir. She subsequently joined the resident choir and her life quality was greatly enhanced by her experiences.

People with dementia live in a world that seems like a 'strange situation' from the onset of symptoms. Miesen (1993) conducted a large-scale series of studies in which he examined the relationship between levels of cognitive functioning, attachment behaviours and parent fixation. Results showed that people with dementia demonstrated similar organized forms of attachment behaviours that Ainsworth (1978) found in her study of infants' attachments to their mothers.

These attachment behaviours were dependant on the various stages of dementia. Parent fixation was common in people with severe dementia (Miesen, 1993). This important study sheds light on our understanding of how to help people with dementia who demonstrate attachment behaviours during the course of their disease. Active music-making as well as passive music listening can become a creative vehicle of safety and security for people with dementia. Adjusting to this theoretical understanding from the carers' perspective offers hope and motivation for coping with each stage of the disease.

Case study

One lady carer attended counselling in order to understand and cope with her husband who had early dementia as well as her own depressive illness. During the course of our conversations, we found a song that helped her to express her confused feelings towards her husband and this improved their relationship. Through the song lyrics and a well-known melody she was able to re-frame her perceptions and deal with past relationship issues that were impacting on her ability to care for her husband in the most appropriate way. These insights also helped her to understand herself and her husband in a more positive light.

Existential theory

Spinelli (1997) believed that a therapist must be prepared to fully enter into a client's present experience: being **with** and for them. Each interaction becomes a here-and-now process in which a trusting and safe environment can develop where the client feels held and protected. Music-making is ideally suited to this philosophy as it meets the person with dementia in the present moment; a moment of deep connection and communication which can engender the emergence of the true 'self' that becomes hidden behind the dementing process.

Laing referred to a splitting of the self into a 'mind'(inner) and a 'body'(outer) in which the individual can identify him/herself more exclusively with the unembodied inner self. When a person is unable to communicate in the ordinary way because of dementia, music therapy can stimulate and awaken the true inner self. Intuitive connections to body language and vocal utterances help to make a connection in which the inner self can be given authentic expression and the person with dementia feels validated.

Yalom (2008) asserted that we 'become who we are' and 'that which does not kill us makes us stronger' (p. 104). Yalom believed that this philosophy was related to activating the client's in-built, self-actualizing forces in order to bring coherence to life.

Case study

An elderly woman in a hostel claimed she had been assaulted by a staff member. My task was to investigate her allegations and facilitate her process after identifying the source of her assertions. She had been abandoned and abused as a young child and this unresolved issue had hindered her psychological growth, leading to bouts of psychotic depression and projections onto others. By listening to a music-based relaxation CD, counselling, poetry and a creative life review, she was able to re-frame her early childhood issues and find something positive and meaningful in her current life without having to remain focused on her traumatic early history.

Singing as the central core of music therapy in dementia care

Singing is represented here as the most potent communicative and musical tool available to people with dementia. We all have a voice and this can be transformed into a creative communicative device when ordinary speech fails. 'The arts are not drugs. They are not guaranteed to act when taken. Something as mysterious and capricious as the creative impulse has to be released before they can act' (E. M Forster cited in Sacks, 2007, p. 299). Singing is a potent channel through which the creative impulse can find expression and release.

Austin (1999) believed that singing can connect a person to breath, physicality and emotion. As people with dementia often experience a sense of disconnection with parts of the self, singing can be a valuable avenue for bringing about a sense of coherence. Austin believed that parts of the self are projected onto the voice and that this type of singing experience could lead to integration of body, mind and spirit.

Music therapy in dementia is not only person-centred but also process-oriented and focused on the present moment. This matches states of awareness and cognitive functioning at various stages of the disease. Helping people with dementia to be silent can produce a state of relaxation and increased awareness. Meditations are effective in producing more positive and relaxed mind-states. Mindell asserted that 'chronic symptoms are like koans, i.e., apparently unanswerable questions meant to increase our consciousness and many such symptoms require dropping our everyday thinking and using awareness to perceive the force of silence in our bodies' (Mindell, 2004, p. 5). Learning awareness through moments of silence can greatly enhance personhood when working with people who have dementia.

Clair (2000) described how elderly people are reluctant to sing because they believe that they do not have a satisfactory voice quality due to the ageing process and early childhood negative responses to their singing. However, once these obstacles are overcome, elderly people find great joy in singing together and achieving a higher level of competence than they thought was possible. This can result in increased motivation, empowerment and social involvement.

I conducted a pilot study (Robertson-Gillam, 2008a) followed by a randomized controlled trial (Robertson-Gillam, 2008b) to investigate whether singing in a choir could reduce depression in people with dementia. Participants became more confident, motivated and communicative. They began to recognize each other and relate meaningfully, reducing levels of social withdrawal that are commonly understood as typifying the dementing process. They made new friends with others living in different residences. They became focused and worked hard to produce the best sounds that they could. They were proud when they were able to participate in performances. However, many choir members asserted that they could not sing properly. This was primarily due to early childhood experiences in which they were told that they did not have a good voice quality. They grew more confident and happier with their voices over time which enhanced their choir membership, sense of belonging and increased life purpose.

Brown et al. conducted a study using singing as a therapeutic caregiving intervention with a group of people in the later stages of dementia. They found that singing during activities of daily living decreased agitation and violent behavioural responses in people with dementia. According to these authors, 'it converts any caregiving interaction into a potential music-making situation' (Brown et al., 2001, p. 36). Many professional and family carers have found that singing while washing, feeding or going for walks has enhanced these activities.

Bannan and Montgomery-Smith (2008) conducted a pilot study where they applied group singing for people with Alzheimer's disease and their carers. They concluded that it is possible for people with Alzheimer's disease to participate in group singing and that some longer-term benefits were perceived by their carers.

Sacks (2007) mentioned the case of Dr P for whom singing was so important that he described his life as one 'that consisted entirely of music and singing'(p. 343). Sacks believed that for people with dementia 'music is no luxury to them but a necessity, and can have a power beyond anything else to restore them to themselves, and to others, at least for a while' (p. 345).

Lester and Petocz (2006) conducted a study with four participants who had dementia, aged between 80–97 years, using singing as a means to reduce the symptoms of disorientation and agitation frequently displayed in the evening hours. Results showed a marked improvement in mood and socialization as well as a significant decrease in non-social behaviour.

Nugent (2002) reviewed 19 music therapy articles which addressed the use of music therapy for reducing agitated behaviours in people with dementia. She found that the literature reviewed *did* support the idea that music therapy interventions were efficacious in reducing agitation in people with dementia.

These studies all demonstrate how the power of the singing voice along with music-making can significantly improve a person's life when they are living with dementia. The creative and spontaneous nature of music is ideally suited to match the state of mind of a person with dementia who lives mostly in the present moment but whose potent memories are from the past. The positive emotional impact of singing and music-making can accumulate over time.

The social effects of choir singing

Being part of a choir helps to increase attention and reduce agitation. In a choir pilot study (Robertson-Gillam, 2008a), many people exhibited agitation and anxiety when they first arrived into the room. Over time, they became more relaxed with increasingly focused attention.

Case study

One lady in the choir always settled down if she could sing a particular hymn called 'Love with Everlasting Love' as the first song. She sang it with much feeling and was able to hold the melody line while I sang the alto part. After that, she could participate in all the other choir activities and remembered some choir events for days after practices.

Case study

Arthur (not his real name) was a physically strong gentleman who had severe dementia. He attended choir practice every week. His attention span was extremely limited and it took a lot of effort on my part as choir leader to keep him engaged. I observed that he manifested agitated behaviours with foot stamping and tearing at the song book. I recognized that Arthur had been a company director and wanted to 'direct' the activity. I encouraged him to help with conducting. He often went to the piano when I was playing and was able to join in, feeling important and validated. A mutual relationship of trust developed between us and his agitation decreased markedly.

Connecting through the Singing Voice in late-stage dementia

Sartre asserted that 'death becomes the meaning of life as the unresolved chord is the meaning of the melody' (Sarte,1966, p. 681). He believed that death is the final boundary of human life and influences the entire life by a reverse flow. 'If the meaning of our life becomes the expectation of death, then when death occurs, it can only put its seal upon life' (p. 683). A diagnosis of dementia has a limiting threshold on life expectancy. This is often a heavy burden for the newly diagnosed person as well as their loved ones as they all struggle to come to terms with the ramifications of the disease. By understanding this philosophy, carers can encourage their loved ones to live their lives more fully in the moment and find many positive events to focus on.

Sacks believed that even in the later stages of dementia when so many other ways of expressing the inner self are stripped away by the disease process, 'there is still a self to be called upon ... even in the face of severe and debilitating cognitive decline ... even if music, and only music can do the calling'(p. 346). For those in the late stages of dementia, music could well be a necessity, even if they have never been previously perceived as musical.

Ansdell (1995) described the extraordinary impact of the singing voice on a patient, Mr G., who was in a coma following a stroke. The music therapist used vocal improvisation as a means of connecting with Mr G., resulting in his eventual recovery. He described his experience as being on a battlefield and that everyone was trying to kill him until he heard the music which he thought was some medieval wind instrument. However, the second time, he did recognize the music as a *voice* and realized that there was someone out there who didn't want to kill him. He felt that 'the music was my music. I decided to live when I first heard the music' (Ansdell, 1995, p. 63).

Case study

Betsy (not her real name) was in the late stages of dementia and had lost the ability to communicate verbally. She regularly wandered up and down the corridor of the nursing home, vocalizing like an opera singer loudly and constantly. I joined her walk one day and matched the pace of her steps. As our rhythm became synchronized, Betsy looked at me and smiled. She sang a wordless phrase to me and I answered her back, mirroring and validating her vocal expression. She listened carefully and we walked on. Then, she sang another musical phrase but extended it from the first one. I answered her back once more and extended the phrase further. She nodded and smiled.

We walked the length and breadth of the nursing home together, singing back and forth. Betsy became more and more reflective and attentive, nodding and saying, 'yes, yes'. Finally, after some time, she stopped and turned to me with a beautific smile on her face. She put her arms around my neck and touched her forehead to mine. We stood like this for some moments and she nodded, saying 'good'. She then walked away, no longer singing but very content. Betsy lived her note, expressing herself through it. She just needed someone to recognize her innate self and she was satisfied.

A note lives, like *you*, like *me*, like them, like *it*.
Moves, stretches and contracts.
Metamorphoses, gives birth, procreates, dies, is reborn.
Seeks, stops seeking, finds, loses.
Marries, loves, tarries, hurries, comes and goes. (Stockhausen, 1968, cited in Boyce-Tillman, 2000)

Musical expression, such as wordless singing and vocalizing, can transcend normal waking reality and meet a person with dementia in the moment. Our voices can express our emotions and recall the song of the soul.

Case study

Bert (not his real name) was agitated, verbally abusive and whistling constantly. He was in the late stages of Alzheimer's disease. Staff found his agitated behaviour disturbing because, no matter what they did to help him, Bert was not comforted.

I sat silently beside him and held his hand. 'C'mon, c'mon' he said loudly. A few times, he swore. I synchronized to his irregular and fast breathing patterns and waited. He whistled as if calling for someone. During his working life, Bert had been a taxi driver and this whistling behaviour could have been a reflection of those days when people would whistle for a taxi. I sang back his musical phrases to him. His whistling seemed pure and clear, like a bird's song.

Bert listened carefully to my vocal mirroring of his whistled messages. After a short pause, he whistled back and I answered the same phrase with vocals. He nodded and whistled a longer phrase, just like Betsy did with her singing. Each time, the musical phrases of whistling and vocalizing became longer and more complicated in their rhythmic and melodic patterns. He stopped and looked at me, smil-ing. He said, 'yes, that's right. You're doing a good job'. I hummed to him while holding his hand and he gradually relaxed and went to sleep for the first time, much to the staff's amazement.

We worked together for six months until Bert was dying. His song which I created was about 'flying away like a bird in the sky'. It became his safety valve as he went through the dying process. In his last session, just six days before his death, he asked me to sing 'up' meaning the bird song and was immediately reassured and com-forted as he related eagerly, deeply and meaningfully with his eyes and body language. Bert touched my life in such a deep way. He was never a person with dementia to me. Bert was a man with a rich life history behind him and the creative task of dying ahead of him. It was the 'bird in sky song' that helped him to fly away.

The connections that were made with Betsy and Bert were deeply moving and meaningful. Both people indicated that their primary communicative modality was a musical one and this needed to be answered with the same language. I believe that music in this way can be like a higher form of communication, even though we may not fully understand what is being communicated.

People in comas are not dissimilar to the mind-states of people in the later stages of dementia. Frequently, the general noise and bustle of a busy nursing home can be confusing for a person with dementia which may have the potential to induce agitated and chal-lenging behaviours. Singing on the other hand, can offer a soft, per-sonal element which leads to deeper engagement with a validating and calming influence.

Conclusion

Music therapy in dementia care is a valuable tool for enabling communication and increasing quality of life. Many studies have been carried out over the past few decades which point to the incredible power of music and singing for reaching and validating people with dementia who experience their lives as *strange* and lose their sense of familiarity with loved ones and the environment. Through music-making, singing and listening, personhood is validated and expressed in the deepest and most meaningful way. People can maintain their essential uniqueness which never dies but can become buried under layers of symp-toms and behaviours that typify the dementing process.

Recent studies in brain plasticity indicate that music has more than entertainment value. They show that music is essential for brain growth and maintenance, providing a safe and therapeutic intervention which can not only increase quality of life but also stimulate brain plasticity and new growth of dendrites for increased cognitive functioning (Cohen, 2006).

All of us as family and professional carers have a voice that we can use for spontaneous vocalizations, and singing of well-known songs as well as playing recorded music to reach, understand and validate the people who live with dementia.

If you are a carer or relative, do not lose heart. Sing to your loved one and listen to their responses. They are still 'there' inside even though the brain mechanism may have broken down, like a television set that has become faulty. The programme is still there but cannot be transmitted adequately. Be patient and immerse yourself in their reality which has become different to yours. By doing this, you will find them again at another level and you will know that love never dies.

For those who are interested in finding out about training in music therapy, courses are available in Australia, Great Britain, United States of America and European countries. The author advises those interested in pursuing a career in music therapy to go online and find relevant courses in their own country. Music therapists must have high musical skills and be aware of the physical aspects concerned in delivering music to disabled people. Furthermore, music therapists are open to the same stressors of transference and counter-transference within the therapeutic relationship that confronts most therapists in the health care industry. Regular mentor supervision is essential to maintain professional and personal standards. Music therapy is better understood in some countries than others so work is needed to raise community and societal awareness of the benefits of this creative approach to dementia care.

References

Ainsworth, M. Blehar, M., Waters, E., & Wall, S. (1978). *Patterns of Attachment.* Hillsdale, NJ: Erlbaum.

Aldridge, D. (1996) *Music Therapy Research and Practice in Medicine: From Out of the Silence.* UK: Jessica Kingsley Press (pp. 186–210).

Aldridge, D. (2005). *Music Therapy and Neurological Rehabilitation: Performing Health.* UK: Jessica Kingsley Press.

Ansdell, G. (1995). *Music for Life: Aspects of Creative Music Therapy with Adult Clients.* UK: Jessica Kingsley Press.

Austin, D. (1999). Vocal Improvisation in Analytically Oriented Music Therapy. In T. Wigram & J. De Baker (eds). *Clinical Applications of Music Therapy in Psychiatry.* UK: Jessica Kingsley Press, 141–158.

Bannan, N. & Montgomery-Smith, C. (2008). Singing for the brain: Reflections on the human capacity for music arising from a pilot study of group singing with Alzheimer's patients. UK. *Journal of the Royal Society for the Promotion of Health,* 128, 2, 73–78.

Benenzon, R. (1992). *Théorie de la musicothérapie à partir du concept de l'ISO.* Bordeaux, France.

Boyce-Tillman, J. (2000). *Constructing Musical Healing: The Wounds that Sing.* UK: Jessica Kingsley Press.

Bright, R. (1972). *Music in Geriatric Care.* Australia: Angus & Robertson.

Bright, R. (1991). *Music in Geriatric Care: A Second Look.* Australia. Music Therapy Enterprises.

Brown, S. (2001). The 'Musilanguage' Model of Music Evolution. In N. L.Wallin, B. Merker and S. Brown (eds), *The Origins of Music.* Cambridge, MA: MIT Press.

Brown, S., Gotell, E. & Ekman, S. (2001). Singing as a therapeutic intervention in dementia care. *Journal of Dementia Care,* July/August 2001, 33–37.

Cabeza, R. (2002). Hemispheric asymmetry reduction in older adults: the HAROLD model. *Psychology and Aging,* 17(1), 85–100.

Christie, M. (1992). Music therapy applications in a skilled and intermediate care nursing home facility: a clinical study. *Activities, Adaptations & Aging,* 16, 69–87.

Clair, A. (1996). *Therapeutic Uses of Music with Older Adults.* Baltimore: Health Professions Press.

Clair, A. (2000). The Importance of Singing with Elderly Patients. In D. Aldridge. (ed.), *Music Therapy in Dementia Care* (pp. 81–101). UK: Jessica Kingsley Press.

Cohen, G. (2006). Research on creativity and ageing: the positive impact of the Arts on health and illness. *Aging and the Arts* American Society on Aging, Spring 2006.

Crystal, H., Grober, E. & Masur, D. (1989). Preservation of musical ability in Alzheimer's Disease. *Journal of Neurology, Neurosurgery & Psychiatry,* 52, 1415–1416.

Cuddy, L. & Duffin, J. (2005). Music, memory and Alzheimer's disease: is music recognition spared in dementia, and how can it be assessed? *Medical Hypotheses,* 64, 229–235.

Fitzgerald-Cloutier, M. (1993). The use of music therapy to decrease wandering: an alternative to restraints. *Music Therapy Perspectives,* 11, 32–36. American Music Therapy Association.

Fukui, H. & Toyoshima, K. (2008). Music facilitate the neurogenesis, regeneration and repair of neurons. Nara University of Education, Takabatake, Nara, Japan. Elsevier Ltd. *Medical Hypotheses.* 71, 5, 765–769.

Gaertner, M. (1999). Sound Of Music in the Dimming, Anguished World of Alzheimer's Disease. In T. Wigram & J. De. Backer (eds), *Clinical Applications of Music Therapy in Psychiatry.* UK: Jessica Kingsley Press, 244–263.

Hays, T. & Minichiello, V. (2005). The contribution of music to quality of life in older people: an Australian qualitative study. *Ageing and Society,* 25, 261–278.

Kenny, C. (1989). *The Field of Play: A Guide for the Theory and Practice of Music Therapy.* Atascadero, CA: Ridgeview Publishing Company.

Kiccolt-Glaser, J., McGuire L., Robles, T. F. & Glaser, R. (2002). Emotions, morbidity and mortality: new perspectives from psychoneuroimmunology. *Annual Review of Psychology,* 53, 83–107.

Lester, B. & Petocz, P. (2006). Familiar group singing: addressing mood and social behaviour of residents with dementia displaying sundowning. *Journal of Music Therapy,* 17, 2–18.

Levitin, D.J. (1994). Absolute memory for musical pitch: Evidence from the production of learned melodies. *Perception and Psychophysics.* 56, 4: 414–423 Levitin & Cook (1996).

Levitin, D.J. & Cook, P.R. (1996). Memory for musical tempo: additional evidence that auditory memory is absolute. *Perception and Psychophysics.* 58, 927–935.

Miesen, B. (1993). Alzheimer's Disease, the phenomenon of parent fixation and Bowlby's attachment theory. *International Journal of Geriatric Psychiatry,* 8, 2, 147–153.

Miller, B., Boone, K., Cummings, J. L., Read, S. L., Mishkin, F. (2000). Functional correlates of musical and visual ability in forntotemporal dementia. *British Journal of Psychiatry,* 176, 458–463.

Miller, B., Cummings, J., Mishkin, F., Boone, K., prince, F. & Cotman, C. (1998). Emergence of artistic talent in FrontoTemporal Dementia. *Neurology,* 51, 4, 978–982. American Academy of Neurology, USA.

Morgan, O. & Tilluckdharry, R. (1982). Presentation of singing function in severe apahsia. *West Indian Medical Journal,* 31, 159–161.

Nugent, N. (2002). Agitated behaviours in Alzheimer's Disease and related disorders: music and music therapy research. Australia. *Australian Journal of Music Therapy,* 13, 38–51.

Odell-Miller, H. (1995). Music Therapy in Psychiatry. In T. Wigram, B. Saperston & R. West (eds), *The Art & Science of*

Music Therapy: A Handbook. Switzerland: Harwood Academic Publishers, 83–112.

Olderog-Millard, K. & Smith, J. (1989). The influence of group singing therapy on the behaviour of Alzheimer's disease patients. *Journal of Music Therapy*, 26, 2, 58–70.

Palmer, M. (1977). Music therapy in a comprehensive program of treatment and rehabilitation for the geriatric resident. *Music Therapy*, 14, 190–197.

Palmer, M. S. (1989). Music therapy in gerontology: a review and a projection. *Music Therapy Perspectives*, 6, 52–56.

Peretz, I., Gagnon, L., Hébert, S. & Macoir, J. (2004). Singing in the brain: insights from cognitive neuropsychology. *Music Perception*, Spring 2004, 21, 3, 373–390.

Robertson-Gillam, K. (2008a). Hearing the Voice of the Elderly. In E. MacKinlay (ed.), *Ageing, Disability and Spirituality*. UK: Jessica Kingsley Press, 163–182.

Robertson-Gillam, K. (2008b). Masters Honours Thesis: *The effects of singing in a choir compared to participating in a reminiscence group on reducing depression in people with dementia*. University of Western Sydney, NSW, Australia.

Sacks, O. (2007). *Musicophilia: Tales of Music and the Brain*. London: Picador Press.

Schneck, D. & Berger, D. S. (2006). *The Music Effect: Music Physiology and Clinical Applications*. UK: Jessica Kingsley Press.

Schoenberger, L. & Braswell, C. (1971). Music therapy in rehabilitation. *Journal of Rehabilitation* [Canada], 37(1), 30–31.

Segal, R. (1990). Helping older mentally retarded persons expand their socialization skills through the use of expressive therapies. *Activities, Adaptation and Aging*, 15(1–2), 99–109 [Special issue: Activities with developmentally disabled elderly and older adults.]

Sixsmith, A. & Gibson, G. (2007). Music and the wellbeing of people with dementia. *Ageing & Society*, 27(1), 127–146.

Spinelli, E. (1997). *Tales of Unknowing: Therapeutic Encounters from An Existential Perspective*. London: Duckworth.

Uddin, L., Molnar-Szakacs, I., Zaidel, E. & Iacoboni, M. (2006). rTMS to the right inferior parietal lobule disrupts self-other discrimination. *Scan*, 1, 65–71.

Winnicott, D. (1971). *Playing and Reality*. London: Routledge.

Yalom, I. (2008). *Staring at the Sun: Overcoming the Dread of Death*. Melbourne, Australia: Scribe Press.

6 Art therapy and dementia care

Patricia Baines

Introduction

Giving me permission to quote his words, a 94-year-old man, who was living with vascular dementia, told me, 'Creativity is of the essence of life. If you think about it, all life is creative.'

I asked another man, in his 80s, who had lived with Alzheimer's disease for some years, what creativity meant to him, and, he said, agreeing that I might share his words,

> I like to be active, to use the old brain box – alive and alert. I feel pretty good after creating something – something achieved.

The point is that individuals living with dementia still retain their desire to be part of a creative world and to express themselves as creative beings. They may be blunter, more honest, perhaps trimmed down of some or even, much of the status-related persona – but when one engages with a person living with dementia, one meets a person living in that precise moment of time and in an intense intimacy of communication.

If she or he is treated as an object or without the capacity to feel, the person living with dementia may comment in one way or another on the failure to recognize her or his humanity. 'All those dark suits walking by. Never even spoke to us,' Violet said with her sense of having been affronted very clear in her voice. The Board of the residential aged care home had passed through the dementia unit without greeting the residents. Interestingly the memory of being ignored had remained.

Simone de Beauvoir, in her classic book on ageing, written almost 40 years ago now, documented the ways in which Western cultures have disparaged and negatively stereotyped those who live to grow old. Ageing women – when 50, and later 60, were considered very old – were often regarded as ugly, and, possibly, dangerous, and old men as foolish and impotent. It is against such a background that the growing reassessment of the rights and creative needs of those, who are growing older and living with dementia, must be set. 'We have not made the life of the aged meaningful or in any sense self-sufficient' (1972, p. 608), de Beauvoir concluded. She spoke of the way the elderly were accommodated in isolation from their successors, with their sense of worth radically reduced after retirement, and their right to participate in decision-making often removed.

The concerns that de Beauvoir felt are reflected in the recent writings of her compatriot, Marie de Hennezel. In her beautiful and inspiring work, *The Warmth of the Heart Prevents Your Body from Rusting* (2008) she seeks to describe how we may learn to age well. Drawing on Gineste-Marescotti's 'philosophy of humanitude', de Hennezel envisages interactions with individuals living with dementia that are intimate and tender and support a sense of worth. She also asks the vital question, 'Can we learn at sixty, seventy, or eighty to liberate our buried creativity if we have not done so earlier in life?' (p. 170). Her answer is an emphatic 'It is never too late to develop our creativity.'

Half a world away in Australia, modest efforts are now being made to involve individuals with dementia living in residential aged care facilities, as well as those still living in the community, in making choices about how they wish to fill their days and to offer them meaningful things to do. Participation in an art therapy group, in which each person is offered acceptance, the right to be heard and the possibility of being creative is one such choice.

Alzheimer's Australia, which is part of a worldwide body, Alzheimer's International, seeks to understand the global prevalence of dementia, to support research into its prevention and find a cure and to educate societies about a person-centred approach to care. For Dementia Awareness month in 2007, the national focus of Alzheimer's Australia was on the value of creative therapies, especially art therapy, to individuals living with dementia.[1]

The premise on which this chapter is based is the belief that all human beings are creative and that being creatively engaged is a human need. When the need to write, paint, dance, sing or make music is met, the person feels a sense of well-being. People living with dementia, enjoy creative expression, even if the means for doing this may need support. Individuals with dementia want to live their lives as fully as possible and desire meaningful activities and genuine interactions. Of course they need to feel safe, warm and comfortable, but life needs to have moments of activity and challenge, moments of achievement and satisfaction.

The chapter will begin by considering the findings of recent research on adult brain plasticity and the value of creative activities to individuals living with dementia. It will then consider the ways in which art therapy can offer a means to resolve grief, anxiety and other issues, which may have pre-existed the diagnosis or be a response to being diagnosed with a disease, which currently has no cure. The last part of the chapter will discuss how one may engage the creativity of individuals living with dementia. The names used in the text are pseudonyms, unless I have been asked to use the real name. I especially thank Jeanne and her family for giving permission to share her images.

Research into the value of creativity

Dementia is the umbrella term for a range of symptoms, which may include short- term and/or long-term memory loss, temporal and spatial disorientation, personality changes, problems with word-finding and so on. The most prevalent neurological diseases, which result in dementia are Alzheimer's disease and vascular dementia (caused by cardio-vascular problems and disease). These are, however, only two of what is sometimes cited as some 50 or of even 70 diseases which cause dementia. Although currently much research is being undertaken globally to understand the causes of the neurological damage and disease, which results in dementia, these diseases remain incurable conditions. The medications, which are currently available, may slow down the process of decline in brain functions for some individuals, but not effect a cure. Whilst dementia has been considered to be a disease of the later years of life (although not part of the normal ageing process), there is a growing number of Baby Boomers (so the under 65s) being diagnosed with Younger Onset Dementia.

What art therapy offers to individuals living with dementia is a therapeutic process, which transcends the limitations of the 'talking' therapies and allows the possibility of resolving psychological issues through various kinds of image-making (with or without words). Rappaport provides another helpful explanation, 'Art therapy incorporates visual art, creative process, and psychotherapy to enhance well-being – emotionally, cognitively, physically, and spiritually' (2009, p. 64).

The most common responses to a diagnosis of dementia are grief, anger and anxiety. The fact that one is also growing older, as well as having a progressive neurological disease, may add a sense of worthlessness through a loss of self-esteem to these initial, normal, responses.

'I'm hopeless,' one elderly man said repeatedly, 'My head's empty.'

'I can't do anything,' an older woman declared, 'I'm useless.'

The art therapist must empower individuals, who have lost confidence in their own creative abilities to begin to make marks again, and, through the creative process, to re-establish a sense of self-worth. Yet the therapeutic purpose of art therapy with individuals living with dementia is also to create a place and space where it is possible to speak about the most dreadful things one is able to imagine.

'What if my children have inherited the disease?' I am asked by a courageous woman with Younger Onset Dementia, who knows that there were family members with dementia in the two preceding generations.

'What if I can no longer recognise my wife?' a man, living with vascular dementia, who repeatedly declares his abiding love for the woman he married, asks with tears in his eyes, but yet so determined to speak the unspeakable.

'The continuation of imagination and engagement provides intervals of good feeling in the face of overwhelming adversity,' concludes Professor Gene D. Cohen (2006), referring to the way group creative activities may be of value to individuals living with Alzheimer's disease. Cohen, whose name is associated with the phrase 'potential beyond problems' and 'positive ageing', has been a long-time advocate of the value of creative activities for older people, including those living with dementia. The words of Dreifuss-Kattan, which are cited by Brosh (2008, p. 235), are also relevant here, 'Writing [*or drawing and painting*] about the fear and pain of loss is itself a process of accepting and overcoming these emotions.' Dreifuss-Kattan used the concept of 'psychological self-repair' to describe what occurs when individuals engage in creative endeavours to face and engage with incurable diseases. The disease may be incurable but emotional, social and spiritual well-being may be achieved alongside and with a progressive illness.

Since 2001, Cohen has been the primary researcher in the Creativity and Ageing Study. This multi-site American study, which involved 3 groups of 50 participants of over 65 (median age 80), taking part in 'professionally-run participatory art activities', with 3 control groups of 50 matched participants, who have continued with their usual activities, is reporting results, which support the value of participating in group art programmes. In the *Final Report* (2006) on the research findings of the project, the researchers conclude, 'The significance of the art programmes is that they foster sustained involvement because of their beauty and productivity. They keep the participants involved week after week, compounding positive effects being achieved.' The effects that were noted in the groups actively participating in creative art activities were: stabilization of overall health, fewer visits to the GP, less medication, fewer falls and improvement on the depression assessment.

Although not specifically described as art therapy, which underlines the importance of the act of creating an image, Cohen did note the importance of participation in a social event. Interestingly, these findings support the research carried out in England by Rusted et al. (2006) into the long-term benefits of art therapy to individuals living with Alzheimer's disease, who noted that participation in art therapy sessions improved mood and alleviated depression.

The research of Cohen and his associates is of particular interest as they seek to understand the reasons why even limited chances to participate actively in various kinds of artistic and creative expression in a group setting are beneficial to health and well-being. Cohen's assertions about the mature brain are based on research findings, which have undone previous beliefs about the brain of the older person. Whilst it was once maintained that the human brain gradually lost neurons and became less and less able to function (so a thesis of gradual brain shrinkage and inevitable decline), research over the past 20 years has instead established that, given the right conditions, the adult human brain continues to develop new brain cells and neural pathways (what is referred to as 'neurogenesis'), and, that the adult human brain demonstrates plasticity. In his book *The Mature Mind* (2005) Cohen identifies four 'key attributes' of the human brain, which offer grounds for a more positive view of growing older, namely: 'The brain is continually resculpting itself in response to experience and learning. New brain cells do form throughout life. The brain's emotional circuitry matures and becomes more balanced with age. The brain's two hemispheres are more equally used by older adults (pp. 3–4).

Cohen's findings are supported by a growing body of research into brain plasticity. Doidge (2007/2010) has provided a skilful overview of this research in his brilliant and readable, *'The Brain that Changes Itself'*. Drawing together the work of Luria, Bach-y-Rita, Merzenich and many other researchers, Doidge states, 'Research has shown that neuroplasticity is neither ghettoized nor confined to the sensory, motor, and cognitive processing areas … it is the property of all brain tissue' (p. 97). What this means, Doidge explains, is that when parts of the brain are damaged or destroyed, other brain tissue may take over to execute the tasks performed by it.

These research findings radically alter the expectations that should be made of older people, even when living with dementia, since, provided with the right conditions, there is the possibility of, at least, partial recovery and of some possible brain renewal. Drawing on these new understandings about the ageing brain, Cohen also suggested that all forms of artistic expression were particularly suitable for older individuals as they optimize the increasing integration of left- and right-brain capacities.

So far, we have established that the older brain may benefit from creative activities, as they support the ways in which the brain continues to develop and change. An environmental condition was, however, suggested in the preceding discussion. Recent research in Brazil carried out as part of the 10/66 studies of the prevalence and forms of dementia in the developing world provided a human comparison to existing animal studies into the effects of impoverished and stimulating/enriched environments. It had been established in laboratories that monkeys and rats brought up in enriched environments developed more neural pathways, than those in environments deprived of stimulation. Johansson (2004:) stated, 'Many studies have shown that an activity-stimulating environment has multiple effects on the brain, including increasing the number of neuronal connections.' The Brazilian study found that environmental factors, which included socio-economic status, which affected access to adequate nutrition as well as to educational opportunities, influenced future risk of dementia. The study suggested that those who lived in poverty may be at greater risk of dementia in later life.

The challenging finding of the Brazilian research is, however, supported by another area of research, namely that which is concerned with brain reserve. Valenzuela and Sachdev (2007, p. 1015) offer a definition of brain reserve as 'a property of the central nervous system related to complex mental activity, which may mediate the course and clinical expression of brain injury'. Following an artistic pursuit as well as playing a musical instrument are two of the categories of complex mental activity. The two researchers had reported in 2006 that individuals who had throughout their lives engaged in complex mental activity showed a 'halved dementia incidence'. The brain reserve proposition is used to explain why individuals, whose brains after their deaths showed definite evidence of neurological damage, did not display the symptoms of dementia when alive. Valenzuela and Sachdev, like the Brazilian study, looked at the value of complex mental stimulation across the lifespan, not just as one grows older.

Drawing together some of these research findings, one must ask whether the mental activity offered in an art therapy group not only alleviates social isolation and low self-esteem, thus ameliorating mood and reducing depression, but also offers meaningful and pleasurable mental activity. Offering an enriched environment may support and enhance the survival of newly formed neurons, and thus, whilst not healing the damaged parts of the brain, may nonetheless offer ways for the brain to transcend disease and find self-expression. In his book, which brings together the findings of his ongoing research, Valenzuela (2009) reviewing the literature about the effects of mental training on the rate of cognitive decline says, 'Mental training of one sort and another tends to slow the rate of cognitive decline over time' (p. 166).

Creating images in the space between: examples of good practice

Serena talked endlessly but her sentences were often incomplete and the turns of phrase unusual. In the midst of her usual flow of partly coherent words, as staff were discussing aloud plans for the dementia unit, in which she lived, Serena turned to me, and asked, 'How will they know what we want if they never ask?'

Lucy also usually spoke in part sentences, sometimes reciting numbers. Asking her permission to write her words down, which she surveyed intently, she suddenly said, 'I've got nothing to do.' The lack of meaningful social activity is not a rare complaint of those living with dementia.

I have never met anyone living with dementia with no memories, or, if denying the presence of memories, at least images or pictures in her or his head. It may sometimes be a challenge to help someone bring the images or words into the space between us. And it is in the space between us that we each place images to create a bridge of understanding. I might offer a figurine or a word in the space immediately before my interlocutor; she or he may look at it, reach out and touch it, respond by using a pen or making marks, using words or expressions. When the spoken word fails, sometimes the sung word is acceptable, when words fail, touch may be the means through which we meet each other. It may be the touch of a mother for a child (and sometimes I am the mother and sometimes the child), of old friends reunited, of giggling school girls holding hands or the respectful shaking of hands. For art therapy is above all else a way to join and be with the person living with dementia, to acknowledge a common humanity, an essential closeness of all beings as we reach out gently and with compassion. Having created a sense of togetherness, it may be possible, indeed often is possible, to address the psychological issues, which are of concern.

Case study

'They say dementia's bad but there are worse things,' Jeanne says to me one day, as she completed a triumphant image of blossoming plants beside a pond, which has reeds like eyelashes around it.

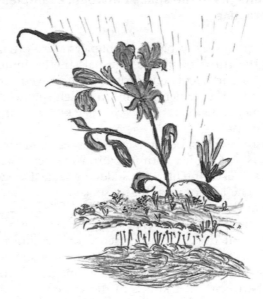

Jeanne's image of growth and flourishing plants

Jeanne, who is in her late 70s, has been and is living with a diagnosis of Alzheimer's disease. Jeanne's images made with intense concentration and interest have become a visual documentation of her changing feelings about her disease and her ability to state that, on reflection, her situation is not as terrible as she first thought.

Jeanne's first image was an unforgettable one of a person in an extraordinary costume of pantaloons and a top with puffed sleeves, with a flag coming out of the head. Jeanne and I both admired the flag, and Jeanne said she had no idea why she had drawn it but it felt right (perhaps expressing her sense of being labelled). The image was accepted and a series of images followed of old trees with broken-off branches and hollowed-out trunks. Jeanne was part of an art therapy group, where others living with dementia spoke about how they coped, of their hopes and fears, and shared their paintings or poems. Slowly, over months, Jeanne's images began to change. She added a few bright autumn leaves to her trees, and, one day, she drew an elderly woman leaning on a walking stick alongside an ageing tree.

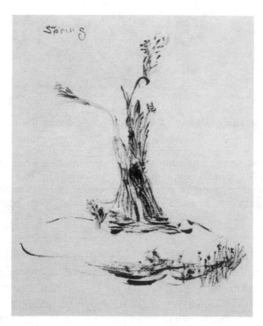

Jeanne's tree begins to show signs of blossoms and a pond is intimated

Over successive months the images continued to change. Water began to appear in the images, then grass and flowers. There was a phase when fish appeared and then gradually the images blossomed that were full of swirls and curls – images that reminded one of the glory of the legendary hanging gardens of Babylon. Jeanne indeed lives with dementia but she now also lives with a sense of her own worth restored. It is not an absolute state but one that needs tending and supporting as her medical condition worsens. Jeanne has also discovered her capacity to reach out and support others with dementia. She now facilitates the creativity of other members of the group by offering ways to begin and encouragement of the first, halting efforts at drawing.

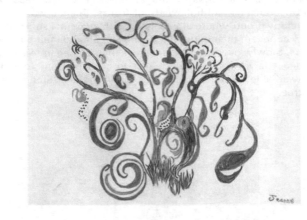

A recent image of Jeanne's – she now facilitates the creativity of others

The activities that happen in the creative space are not a diversion or a time-filler but the substance of meaningful life. To express oneself whether in marks or words, in whatever form, is to participate and communicate. Images are, as the American sculptor, J. Seward Johnson stated, 'declarations of being' (cited by Creek, 2005, p. 81).

Some years ago when displaying the work produced by a group of individuals living with advanced dementia, I paused looking at one sheet with only four or five tiny marks. Fearing that the family might be distressed by the image, I hesitated, but then kept faith to the commitment to honour all marks, and, displayed it. The family, who had in an ongoing way been talking with me about the therapy process, were in fact delighted to see that their mother's creative work had been included. This woman, who was living with younger onset dementia and experiencing severe speech difficulties, was best able to express herself by setting up figurines in a sand tray. Choosing babies, a super woman figure, animals and so on, she made impressive and very articulate communications (I learned to photograph these temporary creations and display these too). Her involvement in the display of art works was, however, important as it was an acknowledgment of her creative presence in the group. The modest exhibition offered recognition of the creative endeavours of those living with dementia in a dementia unit and was a step towards making it a 'more enhancing and nurturing environment' (Junge, 2007, p. 50).

The therapist has the possibility of using the images as a point of dialogue by adding new images.

Case study

A woman in her mid-90s in the late stages of Alzheimer's disease took a baby figurine and showed me birds pecking it. In the context of her few words about older brothers and of being hurt, the possibility of sexual abuse crossed my mind. It was not possible to talk this through in words with her. Instead, I sought to get in touch with the underlying emotion and sense of the image. I offered her tiny dogs to defend and protect the baby. She accepted my suggested solution with a laugh, and, with evident satisfaction, used them to chase away the birds. I cannot say for sure that I had interpreted the situation correctly. Her current environment was a difficult one as other female residents, who did not have dementia, or, not such advanced dementia, showed considerable hostility towards her, but, I had recognized a small child in danger and had offered an idea as to how 'birds' might be dealt with. It did not matter that the elderly woman would probably not remember our interchange. Rather in that moment of image-making, a question had been raised and a symbolic solution discovered.

In the advancing stages of dementia issues may be raised and sorted symbolically across time; that is, not all questions are forgotten. The creative activity continues alongside, perhaps prompting, certainly supporting, the thoughts of concern.

Case study

In her late 90s Regina made drawings of trees and flowers, animals and birds, mixing colours skilfully together and expressing satisfaction at the results. As she worked over some months she discussed a key concern, told me an important dream and finally her resolutions of the question she was asking, which I understood to be about her own mortality and her future beyond that. 'Will my father be coming for me soon?' Regina had asked. 'Will my mother and father be here today? I want to go home,' she spoke softly but her voice was filled with a sense of longing.

The yearning for home is very often part of the later stages of dementia. To answer that her parents were dead would not answer the evident need, instead Regina was offered declarations of affection, reassurances that she was safe and that good parents always knew where their children were, from all those caring for her. By the time I next came to do art therapy with Regina, she told me that she would have to wait a while to go home as the house was being renovated, 'It's a bit worn out and shabby,' she confided (I wondered whether she felt like that about her own body). She grew tired and another resident with dementia came and worked with her on an image of a bird in flight. They enjoyed working together.

Another fortnight had passed, and Christmas Day (so a celebration of a birth) had come and gone. We agreed that Regina would just colour in a part of an image as she said she was very tired. She selected a corner with a flower. As she worked, Regina whispered that she wanted to share something with me. 'I don't know whether it really happened or was a dream. I went on a plane and when I got there, Mum and Dad were there and there was this baby boy and we all held him and we were so happy.' Regina glowed with joy as she spoke. Another fortnight passed. 'One day I'll go to heaven, won't I?' Regina asked, although it was a statement rather than a question.

Across months, Regina had explored ideas about an afterlife, which for her was a going home, to a place where she would be safe and welcomed. Such drawings or paintings, which accompany a search for meaning, may be, as in Regina's case an expression of a conviction of beauty and goodness, or may more frankly explore the underlying issue. Regina had across time carried out her own grief work regarding her mortality. Using the art therapy group as the safe space in which to talk about her reflections and dream work, she had been able to achieve a symbolic resolution; that is, an acceptance of her approaching death.

Case study

A survivor of the Second World War, despite three plane crashes in which he was wounded but never mortally, Osborne made a series of images about ships going down. At the time he was living with both Alzheimer's disease and a terminal illness. He made images of gang planks coming out over the ocean, which might offer an escape route; however, the heaving waves he had painted or drawn were full of sharks and other sea monsters. There was a series of pictures. In one of the later ones Osborne made an arm coming down out of the sky. 'That could be God's arm,' I suggested carefully. My interlocutor roared with laughter and nodded.

Drawing or writing poetry may be a way to assert one's worth against the odds, against a progressive illness, which may take away skills and self-expression. There is a joy in being in a company in which one receives unconditional acceptance. The down side of such closeness is the knowledge of when members of the group go into permanent residential care or die. The group members recall with fondness their memories of the missing person. There is laughter about the quirky or amusing things the person used to say or do. The knowledge, that none of us live forever, is part of the matter-of-factness of group conversation.

Practical guidance

Creating the space for creativity

> 'We all live with one thing or another,' we might say to each other.
> 'Growing old is challenging.' There is a nod, sometimes a grin, of complicity.
> 'It takes courage to keep going as we get older.' A definite affirmative.
> 'There aren't too many advantages to growing old,' the words are offered thoughtfully, and with conviction.
> I smile and reassure, 'Whatever marks you make, whatever you write will be perfect because it comes from you and is about `you.'
> 'I don't know about that,' someone might retort.
> 'Trust your hand,' I say gently, 'your hand remembers what to do.'

I watch in awe and respect as words and lines and colours find their way on to the paper.

Working in various facilities with individuals living with dementia, I rarely have a dedicated space in which to do artwork and writing (so no 'studio'), but rather must each time reconstitute a good place in which to create. It is helpful to bring bits of the environment into the space, so I might gather some of the opening spring buds, flowers, autumn leaves, plants in pots, and a tray of beach sand, a glass bowl of water to enrich the environment and provide a focus of natural beauty for the group. I also set out tiny figurines, which stand for all the things in the world, which we may have encountered, birds and animals, shells and stones, tiny men, women and children, miniature scents, tiny screwdrivers, cars and so on. The art materials are placed carefully so that each person has something to write with and drawing or painting materials are kept immediately in front of her or him. The tables, which are best joined together to create a group, rather than separated, become the inner space in which we create and interact with one another. I move around from person to person kneeling down beside him or her to be at eye level and not towering over the person.

When a person with dementia has objects available to stimulate the brain, she or he will often (but not always) find that something (an image, an idea) comes to her or him. The basic understanding is that the person with dementia finds it difficult to start from nothing. If I am asked why we have these small objects around us, I explain that, when one has some memory loss, they assist the brain to get started. We use them, not because the person with dementia is a child, but because we need to begin from something. The objects are good to think with. If someone resists what looks like toys, then more obviously adult things, such as a tray of shells or a bowl of water, or a tray of sand and pebbles may be used.

Art therapy is a process which allows individuals, in a space in which they cannot be wrong or make mistakes, to explore through images their hopes and fears and memories. The images may be painted, drawn, made as a collage or by using words. Creating a judgment-free space is critical. It is important to say aloud things like: 'Nothing you do can be wrong.' 'The artist is always right.' 'Whatever marks you make will be right.' It is essential that the participants understand that these, often hesitant and tentative acts of creation, are not to be mocked or laughed at. The therapist must model respect and delight in the creative process and assist group members to see the beauty in words, which are no longer grammatical, but have become a kind of poetry, to wonder aloud at images which reveal something of what it feels like to live with dementia.

Participants laugh in delight at my words about the space: 'This must be the only place on earth where we can't be wrong!'

Tuning the space and warm ups

The difficulty of starting an image may be dealt with in a number of different ways. A very talented ex-teacher with vascular dementia, who lived alone, liked to be given a clutch of sheets with the beginnings of stories on them. She would then use the typed words to start a lengthy story, which she could write when given the starting phrase. Although initially supplying fairly realistic beginning, which allowed for autobiographical material (e.g. 'When I was young, I was happy when …', 'At school I enjoyed…'), I later offered beginnings, which could be used for more imaginative writing ('Long, long ago in a forest…' 'Once upon a time there was a young girl …'). It was possible to teach the daughter of this gifted woman to write beginnings for her mother.

There are obviously many ways to play with words. A silver foil pond can be made on a table and filled with small paper fish, each of which has a word written on it. Words may be elicited from the group by giving a starting word such as 'springtime' or 'earthshine'. A whiteboard or inexpensive paper may be used to record all of the group's responses and then the group may be invited to do something with the words or whatever they have triggered (they need to be visible as with dementia remembering the words is often not possible – the therapist must create a stock of images and words, which do not vanish). Some individuals with dementia, who feel that drawing is difficult, may respond to an invitation to make a collage. Cutting out and glueing skills may be present or, with more advanced dementia, absent, but the therapist can use ready-made images to provide the basis for creative expression. Gardening magazines and the National Geographical, collected from garage sales (car boot sales) and markets, provide inexpensive and effective sources of images. It may be necessary to cut the images out for the person with dementia, some in advance, and others selected by the individual in the session.

It will have become evident that there is a slant to the therapeutic process, in that the offering of positive, life-affirming and healthy images, precedes the expression of negative images. As and art therapist I create not just a safe place but a rich and interesting space, which has signs of a wider and wonderful world. The response to colour and interesting things is strong. 'It's a party' someone says as they enter the space. A man who has previously avoided interaction is drawn in by a large see-through container of coloured pens, 'I thought they were lollies.' The space can be shaped with plants or shells, as well as by talk about some of the beautiful things that have occurred or are occurring – the birth of babies, the growth of new leaves, the discovery of a 34,000-year-old flute of griffon vulture bone. French perfume or sprigs of lavender may open another channel for the imagination.

The therapist then is a kind of tuner of the process, adding images and words, as the group needs them in order to keep being able to produce their own creations, or simply watching and affirming non-verbally and verbally as is appropriate. The therapist must move in a kind of dance between holding the group and relating with individuals very closely and in an immediacy and focus that for a moment actually excludes the rest of the group members. To really be with a person requires proximity and being on a level with the person (not towering over her or him) may require touch as well as face-to-face communication. With individuals living with dementia one cannot smile too often, for smiling is read as the world being happy and well and in order. When the images or words are of terror or anger or grief, the therapist must be with the person in that place and space and then gently assist the person to add to the image to create a way forward or at least a place beside the heavy or dark place.

There are sound neurological explanations for the effectiveness of countering overwhelming negative images with positive images. 'Art therapy may help pair the experience of a new benign image with the memory of old fearful images ... providing positive experiences associated with serotonin release [which] can mediate fear' (Hass-Cohen et al., 2008, p. 296 in Hass-Cohen and Carr [eds]). Supporting positive images, yet not suppressing negative memories, but, creating links between them, to temper the older distressing image, may provide a way forward towards well-being despite living with an incurable progressive disease.

Conclusions and the way forward

Offering individuals living with dementia the opportunity to express themselves creatively, in whatever medium he or she chooses, is to begin to re-establish positive meaning to living. That act of self-expression made in a group setting offers recognition and engagement. That achievement, when faced by an increasingly debilitating disease, is of value in and of itself. Yet as an art therapist working with individuals living with dementia, it has already been necessary to develop ways of working which take cognizance of the damage to the brain. Thus whilst the value of the creative art process is common in all the areas in which art therapy is used, it is clear now from the advances in neurological understanding of adult brain plasticity that art therapists will need to address not only the psychological issues raised by individuals living with dementia, thus the psychotherapeutic dimension of the process, but also plan therapeutic activities and opportunities to enhance and support neurogenesis. 'Where gains reflect plasticity there will be a need to design rehabilitation techniques that have the potential to promote activity in the targeted brain areas and support the recruitment of compensatory circuits' (Clare, 2002, p. 62). Whether imagination can be so particularly focused, or is rather a utilization of many parts of the brain, is a challenging question. Certainly Francis Kaplan, an experienced American art therapist, whom I had the privilege to meet when she came to work at Edith Cowan University in Western Australia, envisaged such a dialogue between neurologists and art therapists. In her introduction to *Art therapy and Neuroscience* she wrote, 'The scientific theory of art therapy must take into account the findings of evolutionary biology and anthropology concerning mankind, and the findings of neuroscience and psychology concerning the workings of the human brain and the findings of the physical sciences concerning the laws of nature.' (p. 94). In the same volume, Hass-Cohen commented on these words and said, 'Art therapy is poised to take advantage of the abundance of information from clinical neuroscience research.'

The plasticity of the brain and its capacity to grow more neurons has overturned the previous thinking that we have a given and finite number of cells in our brains, which, once used up or destroyed, means the end of mental activity. The discussion now revolves rather around the best conditions for neurogenesis and what promotes and allows new neurons to become part of the original brain network. In doing art therapy 'the challenge is to learn enough about the mechanisms of plasticity to be able to guide them, suppressing changes that may lead to undesirable behaviours while accelerating and enhancing those that result in a behavioural benefit' (Pascuel-Leone et al., 2006, p. 315, cited in Hass-Cohen 2007, p. 27). Whilst this is an inspiring and long-term goal for art therapists, creative activities which stimulate the brain seem to offer a hopeful and satisfying way for the individual living with dementia to participate in life. Creative activities practiced in a supportive and therapeutic environment also benefit from 'a minimal potential for harm' (Valenzuela & Sachdev, 2005a).

Note

1. I was invited to write the publication which is part of the Best Practice series and is called 'Nurturing the heart: creativity art therapy and dementia'. It is available online at www. alzheimer's org.au

References

Brosh, H. (2008). Not Being Calm: Art Therapy and Cancer. In M. Liebmann (ed.), *Art Therapy and Anger* (pp. 226–237). London and Philadelphia, PA: Jessica Kingsley Publishers.

Clare, L. (2002). *Neuropsychological Rehabilitation and People with Dementia*. New York: Psychology Press.

Cohen, G. (2005). *The Mature Mind: The Positive Power of the Aging Brain*. New York: Basic Books.

Cohen, G. (2006). Research on creativity and aging: the positive impact of the arts on health and illness. *Generations*, 30(1), 7–15.

Creek, J. (2005). The Therapeutic Benefits of Creativity. In T. Schmid (ed.), *Promoting Health through Creativity* (pp. 74–89). London and England: Whurr Publishers.

De Beauvoir, S. (1972). *Old Age.* Harmondsworth, Middlesex: Penguin.
De Hennezel, M. (2008). *The Warmth of the Heart Prevents the Body from Rusting: Ageing without Growing Old.* Carlton North, Victoria: Scribe.
Doidge, N. (2007/2010). *The Brain That Changes Itself* (Revised edition). Carlton North, Victoria: Scribe Publications.
Hass-Cohen, N., Carr, R. & Kaplan F. F. (2008). *Art Therapy and Clinical Neuroscience.* London and Philadelphia, PA: Jessica Kingsley Publishers.
Johansson, B.B. (2004). Brain plasticity in health and disease. *Keio Journal of Medicine,* 53 (4): 231–246.
Junge, M. B. (2007). The Art Therapist as a Social Activist. In Frances, F. Kaplan (ed.), *Art Therapy as Social Action* (pp. 40–55). London and Philadelphia, PA: Jessica Kingsley Publishers.
Rappaport, L. (2009). *Focus-Oriented Art Therapy.* London and Philadelphia, PA: Jessica Kingsley Publishers.
Rusted, J., Sheppard, L. & Waller, D. (2006). The multi-centre randomized control group trial on the use of art therapy for older people with dementia. *Group Analysis,* 39(4), 517–536.
Scazufca, M., Menezes, P. R., Araya, R., Di Rienzo, V. D., Almeida, O. P., Gunnell, D. & Lawlor, D. (2008). Risk factors across the life course and dementia in a Brazilian population: results from the Sao Paulo Ageing and Health Study. *International Journal of Epidemiology,* 37, 879–890.
Valenzuela, M. J. (2009). *It's Never Too Late to Change Your Mind: The Latest Medical Thinking on What You Can Do to Avoid Dementia.* Sydney, NSW: Harper Collins Publishers.
Valenzuela, M. J. & Sachdev, P. (2005). Brain reserve and dementia: a systematic review. *Psychological Medicine,* 36, 441–454.
Valenzuela, M. & Sachdev, P. (2007). Assessment of complex mental activity across the lifespan: development of the Lifetime of Experiences Questionnaire. *Psychological Medicine,* 37(7), 1015–1026.

7 Applying complementary therapies with a person-centred approach

Kirsten James

Introduction

The way all humans experience and connect with the world around them is impacted by the senses. Complementary Therapies can offer connectedness via the senses, and therefore be a useful and dynamic means by which communication and perception can be enhanced. They can act as a key to 'unlock' memories, feelings, emotions and abilities that may not be apparent.

Dementia complicates the impact of sensory experience by also affecting communication and perception. Therefore the quality of life of those with this condition is undeniably affected. As health professionals and carers, recognizing this and having a repertoire of holistic and person-centred interventions to support the affected person enhances outcomes for both parties.

Although there is no universally agreed definition, the term Complementary Therapies commonly refers to the use of therapies or interventions that can work alongside and in conjunction with (Western) orthodox or mainstream treatments and care, so that a more holistic approach is achieved (NBV Guidelines, 1999; British Medical Association).

Individually tailored Complementary Therapies can help to tap into and nurture the physical, psycho-social-spiritual, emotional, cognitive and cultural care needs of the individual and those close to them. Facilitating two-way communication, creativity and intimacy by stimulating and/or soothing the senses and invoking long-held memories, can mean that daily life of the person with dementia can be improved.

They can also minimize stressors, maximize abilities and reduce behavioural and psychological symptoms of dementia through relaxation (Sierpina et al., 2005). Importantly, they can reduce the need for medications and work alongside and in conjunction with orthodox medical treatment (hence the term 'complementary').

Most importantly, as with any treatment or therapy, they should never be applied in a formulaic fashion, but initiated in accordance with an individual assessment of the person and in consultation with their next of kin (Bird, 2009).

This chapter defines what Complementary Therapies are, outlines how they can enhance care and quality of life of the person with dementia and identifies the practical, professional and political issues that need to be considered for them to be implemented successfully. Examples of good practice will be provided, as well as practical guidance and directions.

Background

Complementary Medicine and Therapies have a long – and in some cases ancient – history in many cultures around the world and in the West and have been subjected to much political debate (McCabe, 2001). The terms alternative, complementary, unorthodox, traditional and natural are often used interchangeably in the media, causing much confusion. However, most practitioners in the field and advocates of these modalities prefer the term Complementary Therapies because they feel that the other terms have negative connotations.

The National Institute of Complementary Medicine in Australia says that the term 'complementary' means 'forming a complete or balanced whole' and states that 'Complementary Medicine (CM) includes a diverse range of medicines and therapies that are not practices or core conventional allied health practices' (NICM, 2009).

The Cochrane Complementary Medicine Field says, 'These practices complement mainstream medicine by 1) contributing to a common whole, 2) satisfying a demand not yet met by conventional practices, and 3) diversifying the conceptual framework of medicine' (Manheimer & Berman, 2007).

A broad range of therapies exist under the banner of 'Complementary and Alternative Medicine (CAM)', from complete health philosophies such as naturopathy, chiropractic, osteopathy, kinesiology, traditional Ayurvedic or Chinese medicine to manipulative, body-based practices such as massage, reflexology, yoga, therapeutic dance, aromatherapy or those of a more psychotherapeutic nature such as pet therapy, doll (or 'Child Representational') therapy or meditation. Energy therapies such as Reiki and Therapeutic Touch are another domain (NICM, 2007).

Although enjoying unprecedented popularity in the general community, Complementary Therapies have been considered controversial. For example, some of these therapies and their practitioners do not have established minimum standards of practice, have not been subjected to evidence-based research, do not have standardized or minimal education requirements nor are subject to regulation by any recognized authority. However, some people are prejudiced against these therapies simply because they do not understand them; many of them operate under a different paradigm to the modern Western biomedical model of health care (e.g. acupuncture as a Traditional Chinese Medicine treatment). These factors result in their being regarded by critics with suspicion and disdain.

This being said, there has been a considerable shift since the 1990s in the West, which has seen increasing research in the field of Complementary Therapies, and the development of academic institutions, regulatory bodies and insurance coverage.

This shift has seen a much wider acceptance and acknowledgement of Complementary Therapies as legitimate and valuable tools in the dementia care repertoire. Although they are not readily available in all community, health and residential care settings, they are certainly more accessible than ever before.

This change is reflective of the current sociopolitical context of aged care that includes the following characteristics:

- Advocacy versus custodial,
- Individual care focus versus collective,
- Person-centred versus task-orientated,

- Multicultural with differing health care paradigms,
- Consumer (or their representative) driven,
- Increased awareness of their rights, more informed, demanding choices,
- Service providers bound by legislation, standards, regulations, accountability,
- Focus on preventative or rehabilitative health care to reduce the cost of care.

There are a number of reasons for the use and increased popularity of Complementary Therapies, and these include

- cultural and traditional beliefs,
- dissatisfaction with modern western medical practices and relationships with conventional doctors,
- improved availability of consumer health information and awareness of individual rights to self-determination and choices,
- the desire to be treated holistically, as a 'whole person' rather than symptomatically,
- 'time, touch and talk' as well as encouragement of patient participation in the Complementary Therapy process,
- increased evidence of the benefits of safety of Complementary Therapies and Medicine. (State Government of Victoria, 2009)

Evidence base

Aims and benefits of Complementary Therapies

Health professionals and carers alike can feel overwhelmed by the negativity of dementia. Viewing dementia as a progressive, degenerative condition that ultimately contributes to the person's demise is unhelpful to the person with dementia. It can also influence how the carer responds and can ultimately lead to premature burnout (Zimmerman et al., 2005).

Focusing on the person's retained senses, skills and abilities is helpful, but these are not always obvious or apparent. They can also vary from day to day, even minute by minute. Being able to mutually connect with the person and tap into the essence or spirit of who the person is now and who they have been in the past, is both constructive and rewarding; '*Looking at the light, rather than the lampshade*' (Trout, 1990).

According to Moyle (2008), the aims of using Complementary Therapies in the dementia care context are

- to positively influence emotional and behavioural changes associated with dementia;
- to enhance remaining skills and to help the person with dementia adapt to life;
- to calm and reduce disruptive behaviours such as aggression and non-aggressive agitation;
- to support caregivers;
- to engage the person in the sensations of living until they die.

Although difficult to measure in this population, because Complementary Therapies help to engage the person with dementia, they can also enhance psychosocial qualities of life, such as feeling cared about and secure.

These are qualities of the positive caring relationship that are often overlooked, and which support the person-centred philosophy of care by providing opportunities for the person with dementia to creatively express themselves and feel acknowledged: Whether it be expression through the touch of massage, petting an animal, the joy of sharing a favourite song or dancing – all are ways of engaging the person as an individual and can be person-led. They are also effective non-verbal means of communication – verbal skills commonly being impacted by dementia.

Complementary Therapies promote 'interpersonal connection' (Taylor, 2001) between the person and their carer, and not only support the maintenance of retained skills but also trigger long-held memories (both negative and positive, so caution is required). They can provide pleasurable sensory experiences and emotional enrichment through the stimulation and/or soothing of the senses. They can provide occupation and leisure to help stave off boredom and isolation.

A wonderful example of this is espoused by Naomi Feil, the founder of Validation Therapy. She promotes the gentle stroking of the temples whilst looking into a person's eyes as a way of invoking the memories of mother-child interaction. In one particular example, she combines this approach with singing favourite music to the lady with whom she is engaging, resulting in her responding when she has been non-verbal for a long time (see www.memorybridge.com).

Other benefits to the person with dementia

> Agitation, stress and increased cortisol production further restricts the functional capacities of patients with dementia.
>
> *Sierpina et al.*

A benefit elicited by a number of Complementary Therapies is what Herbert Benson termed 'The Relaxation Response' (Benson & Klipper, 1977). This response can have significant benefits for anyone, including

- reduced heart rate and blood pressure,
- decreased respiration rate,
- reduced cortisol levels,
- improved digestion,
- reduced agitation,
- decreased pain awareness,
- maintenance of blood sugar within normal range,
- improved memory and decision making. (Benson and Klipper, 1977)

Experiencing something pleasurable involves the stimulation of endorphins – neuropeptides that are similar in effect to morphine and yet are produced by the body naturally (Pert, 1997). Endorphin stimulation can improve mood, promote a sense of calm and relaxation, reduce pain and boost the immune system (Burns, 1996).

The perils of using psychotropic medications in the elderly are well documented, with side effects ranging from increased risk of falls, heart disease and blood pressure irregularities to worsening confusion and agitation, to name a few (Gurvich &

Cunningham 2000). The successful utilization of Complementary Therapies can potentially result in a reduction in the use of psychotropic medications. For example, where a person finds hand massage relaxing, this can be applied to help calm, soothe and reduce their pain by providing a distraction, promoting muscle relaxation, lowering their heart rate and blood pressure and reducing their respiratory rate – all of which are measurable outcomes but rarely used to assess impact of therapy. If they are prescribed analgesia, then they may not require as much of the medication as often if a state of relaxation is successfully induced.

Some of the most common symptoms experienced by people with dementia that can cause or exacerbate their behavioural and psychological symptoms include pain, constipation, anxiety, infection and sleep disturbance (Alzheimer's Australia, 2008).

By promoting relaxation, improving the immune system and reducing the use of psychotropic medication, Complementary Therapies can potentially have a profound impact on improving the person with dementia's quality of life.

Carer benefits

Caring for people with dementia can create many burdens – emotionally, physically, spiritually and financially (Access Economics, 2009). In the education program 'Creative Ways to Care', home-based carers stated that they had an improved sense of satisfaction and sense of connection by learning a range of Complementary and Diversional Therapies with the person they cared for. As one gentleman stated regarding his wife *'It made such a difference to have these skills or tools that I could use to move my wife from a sad to a happy place…. and if she's happy, then I'm happy'* (Commonwealth Respite and Carelink Centre Southern Region, 2009).

If Complementary Therapies are utilized as part of a person-centred approach to care in residential care settings, they can impact on staff satisfaction, retention and the quality of care provided. According to Zimmerman et al. (2005) staff who are able and encouraged to practice person-centred care demonstrated positive attitudes related to their level of satisfaction and perceived competence in providing dementia care.

The cost benefits of reducing organic and behavioural symptoms is an excellent reason for Complementary Therapies to be at least tried preventively (and the result documented) as a care intervention. If carer burden on all levels can be reduced, then there is a higher chance of the person with dementia being able to maintain a stable home environment (whether in care at home or in professional residential care). This element is not only important economically for the individual but also for the community at large.

A stable home environment, with minimal disruptive relocations is also important because such moves are likely to hasten the person with dementia's cognitive decline (Alzheimer's Australia, 2008).

As health professionals and carers of people who are cognitively impaired, it is easy to assume that the caring role is a one-way street, with the person with dementia always being the receiver of what the carer gives. However, providing the person with dementia with opportunities to reciprocate is a powerful and effective way of helping them to feel acknowledged and valued and can enhance the relationship. For example, during a hand massage, the person with dementia can be encouraged to massage the carer's hands in return, providing mutual pleasure, relaxation and connection.

Another benefit from the carer perspective is that by observing the person carefully in any number of these therapies, there is an opportunity to gauge their condition progression in a subtle, non-obtrusive way. For example, noting increased perseveration during particular activities (art, music, pet therapy, hand massage and so on) may indicate worsening of the condition and care interventions can be adapted accordingly (Innes & Hatfield, 2001, pp. 23–29).

Research and Complementary Therapies in dementia

Academics agree that there is a dearth of good quality research in Complementary Therapies in general and in Complementary

Therapies in dementia (Alzheimer's Society UK, 2009; Australian Government, 2008; Dunning, 2006; Moyle, 2008; O'Connor et al., 2009).

Recent literature reviews reveal that encouraging results are evident in the fields of music, exercise, aromatherapy, massage and muscle relaxation (Moyle, 2008; O'Connor et al., 2009). Moyle also concluded that Complementary Therapies in dementia can have mixed effects depending on the person, staff or care environment (2008).

One challenge is the nature and complexity of holistic health care interventions and challenges involved in applying standard research methodology. Taylor writes '... *if I am researching the effectiveness of a complementary therapy it will always be in relation to all aspects of the humans experiencing it, that is, in the context of their biopsychosocial and spiritual wellbeing. Do not separate the therapy from the humans experiencing it and fail to reconnect them*' (McCabe, 2001). One could argue that the underlying philosophical underpinnings of the 'Complementary' approach do not lend themselves naturally to the application of a rigorous scientific method. This being said, the impact of their often subtle, sensitive and complex characteristics are probably best captured qualitatively rather than quantitatively. One should also note that 'expert opinion', although not as strong as other bases, is evidence nonetheless (Joanna Briggs Institute, 2008).

In summary, although further good quality research to date in this field is required, there are clear indications that a range of Complementary Therapies show promise and potential for a positive impact on many symptoms of dementia. Empirical evidence suggests that they clearly offer a number of creative and positive ways for carers to interact and respond to the needs of people with dementia, in keeping with a holistic and person-centred approach, and should not be discounted.

Examples of good practice

The following examples of Complementary Therapies have been chosen because they are familiar to many, are practical and accessible and have been known to have positive impacts on behavioural and psychological symptoms of dementia. It is important to note, however, that one should never 'dabble' in Complementary Therapies, but be well-informed about the therapy utilized.

Clinical Psychologist and researcher in the field of dementia, Mike Bird (2009) notes that the important tenets for guiding the use of different interventions should include

- first, do no harm; always minimize risk and maximize safety,
- be informed about indications and contraindications,
- have policies and procedures in place and
- seek professional advice from suitably qualified persons as required.

Guidelines for choosing a particular therapy should also be contingent on the following:

- Individual assessment of the individual consumer, having regard for their choices and health goals,
- Consultation and consent of next of kin (presuming the person with dementia is not cognitively competent) and sensitivity to the consumer's culture and belief system,
- Available evidence of the safety and efficacy of the therapy based on empirical data and research,
- Education and experience of the health professionals involved,
- Access to professional support, consultation and referral networks,
- Policies and procedures in place, including legal, ethical and quality considerations. (See Appendix 7.1 'Guideline principles for development of policies and procedures', NBV Guidelines, 1999)

Dunning has outlined a clear summary of Clinical Practice Guidelines in the context of Complementary Therapies with a list of examples which is helpful for those seeking to develop their own (2006, pp. 67–72). Guidelines for evaluation are also necessary.

Most suitable therapies for health professionals that require some basic training include environmental manipulation, distraction techniques, music, simple hand or foot massage, simple aromatherapy, the use of simulated or real animals and doll or 'Child Representational' therapy.

However, as stated earlier – awareness of indications and contraindications of each therapy is important, as is individual assessment and consent. Without background knowledge, preparation and guidelines in place, any therapy can yield undesirable results.

With older people, important considerations such as sensory changes, skin condition, metabolism and condition of the physical body (i.e. co-morbidities), possible interactions with prescribed medications, negative memory associations and communication with the health care team and consumer's family need to be addressed prior to introducing any therapy.

Massage

Definition

> Massage is '... a conscious, deliberate, and often formalised use of the instinctive response to comfort another person using touch' (Rankin-Box, 1995, p. 127). It comes from the Greek *masso*, to knead, and the Arabic *mass*, to press gently. (Olsen, 1992)

It is recommended that staff receive competency-assessed basic training in foot and hand massage, but for other areas of the body, a qualified massage therapist is required.

Benefits

Benefits include

- reduction in anxiety levels,
- emotional stress relief,
- relief of muscular tension and fatigue,
- improved circulation and skin integrity,
- enhanced joint mobility,
- pain relief,

- connection/communication between giver and receiver,
- comfort and reassurance.

Contraindications and precautions

Contraindications include infection, acute injury such as open wounds, fractures, haematoma, torn ligaments and severe pain of unknown origin.
Precautions include

- medication – anticoagulants, corticosteroid therapy,
- diabetes – nerve supply, circulation may be affected,
- acute inflammatory conditions – arthritis, gout,
- previous injury or surgery – carpel tunnel, microsurgery, scarring, contractures,
- desensitization and awareness – paralysis, stroke

Case study

Deprivation of touch in older people (for men in particular) is well documented (Bush, 2001; Ebersole et al., 2004). Carl and Wally were residents of a high-care dementia-specific facility. Family visits were seldom, so it was not surprising for care staff to observe how much each enjoyed a regular hand massage. One day, as two staff members were offering hand massage to these gentlemen in the same room at the same time, Wally started to massage the carer's hands. She responded with appreciative sighs, saying how nice it felt. Carl started to do the same with his carer. Broad grins appeared on both gentlemen's faces as the carers responded favourably to the caring touch they were receiving. Through this unexpected reversal of roles, the carers realized the significance of providing caring opportunities for the people that are usually care recipients, providing them with a sense of self-worth.

Aromatherapy

Definition

the controlled use of essential oils from named botanical sources, which are used to assist the body to regulate and rebalance itself. (Dunning, 2007, p. 6)

Benefits

Aromatherapy is especially popular in aged and palliative care, and is most commonly used to

- improve the environment,
- provide sensory stimulation,
- improve sleep,
- improve pain management,
- reduce stress and anxiety,
- enhance appetite and food enjoyment,
- modify behavioural and psychological symptoms of dementia,
- improve communication,
- contribute to the well-being of relatives and carers. (Dunning, 2007, p. 248)
- inhalations of Lavender oil were found to reduce agitation significantly (Holmes et al., 2001); Melissa officianalis (lemon balm) oil was found to reduce agitation when applied to hands and arms twice a day (Ballard et al., 2002).

There are two main ways in which aromatherapy works – through inhalation and skin absorption. Effective inhalation methods that can be used readily for people with dementia include

- vaporization using an approved electric vaporizer placed out of the person's reach,
- drops of essential oil being placed on a tissue or handkerchief, and tucked into the person's day clothing, or pyjamas or pillow at night,
- compresses or scented wash cloths. (see Appendix 7.1)

Essential oils can be absorbed via the skin when they are incorporated into

- baths and foot spas, and also
- creams, gels or carrier oils for massage.

If used in a professional health care context, staff training is important, and at the very least, the involvement of a qualified aromatherapist is advised.

Contraindications and precautions

Responsibilities of individual practitioners and copies of guidelines are outlined clearly by Dunning (2007, p. 85). She also recommends that '... when selecting essential oils for therapeutic purposes health professionals need to take into account the individual's needs, the quality and purity, chemical composition, absorption, distribution and metabolism of essential oils and the various application/administration methods' (Dunning, 2007, p. 135).

Case studies

1. An elderly nun with dementia apparently hadn't spoken for many months. A nurse and qualified aromatherapist was giving the nun a sandalwood foot massage, when the nun spontaneously began talking about going horse riding with her father when she was a child. She recalled the velvet on her riding jacket and the smell of her father's sandalwood aftershave with fondness. Staff were gobsmacked to hear her speaking after such a long time – the aromatherapy providing a communication 'key' effectively unlocking this lady's speech and long-held memories.

2. Staff of a high-care nursing home implemented aromatic wash cloths at mealtimes. This resulted in hygiene needs being met with dignity and minimal stress. The daily ritual acted as a memory cue and promoted appetite stimulation (James, 2006).

3. A cautionary tale: A professional carer attended a weekend aromatherapy workshop. She had learned that camomile essential oil was an effective anti-irritant. Filled with enthusiasm (and limited knowledge) upon her return to work, she applied drops of camomile essential oil into an elderly lady's eye, resulting in a chemical 'burn' and causing pain to the lady. As well as the distress caused to the lady, the organization put a blanket ban on all Complementary Therapies following the incident. The moral of the story is that dabbling can be dangerous!

Pet animal and simulated animal therapy

Definition

Pet therapy usually implies the informal interaction of domesticated animals with humans in either a companion or visiting capacity. Simulated animals can also be used very effectively for people with dementia, and/or in situations where the presence of live animals is not condoned or practical.

Benefits of human-animal interaction that have been identified as a valid experience for people with dementia: Occupation and sense of purpose, Companionship, reducing sense of isolation and depression, Improved socialization and reduced aggression, Opportunity for comfort and nurturing, Source of distraction and promotion of play, Memory stimulus (reminiscence), Promotion of balance, mobility and activity, Reminiscence and relaxation benefits, Case reports and several pilot studies have suggested benefits of pet therapy, but there is limited research to date.

Contraindications and precautions

For both visiting and residential animals the following need to be considered:

- Environment suitability,
- Possible allergies or negative memory associations for people with dementia,
- Costs of feeding, vaccinations and general care,
- Policies to include responsibility of care, infection control issues,
- Protocols for safety, for example visiting dogs on leads, residential pets to not receive supplemented feeds and so on.

Case studies

- Beryl was transferred to a psycho-geriatric assessment facility from a nursing home because of persistent vocalization. She was physically frail and legally blind, and had no family or friends who visited. She often spoke fondly of a pet cat that she had when she was young. An interactive simulated cat was introduced to Beryl which kept her meaningfully occupied as she enjoyed petting, talking to it and holding it in her lap. These interactions helped to reduce her vocalizing for short periods of time and became a useful prompt for reminiscence with volunteers and paid carers who were organized to visit her.
- A 'dementia care farm' has been established at a nursing home on the outskirts of Melbourne, Australia where the Director of Nursing has successfully implemented a small animal farm, with vegetable and herb gardens on site. This is based on a Dutch model of care, where residents are encouraged to interact with the animals through carefully supervised petting as well as helping to care for them.

Doll Therapy

Definition

Doll Therapy is a validation/reminiscence that provides meaning to people with dementia with an opportunity to connect with their caring and parenting instincts through interaction with a 'lifelike' baby doll. The most therapeutic value appears to be achieved when the individual is at a stage in their dementia where they perceive the doll as a real baby (although some people will still gain benefit when they recognize the doll as a doll).

Benefits

This particular therapy can be used successfully to meet the unmet emotional needs and reduce the signs of ill-being of people with dementia such as verbal and physical aggression, wandering, restlessness and anxiety. Specifically, this therapy can

- provide an opportunity for people with dementia to express their emotions;

- provide meaningful communication opportunities through interacting with and talking about the baby doll;
- provide people with dementia a sense of validation, role and purpose by taking care of the baby doll;
- provide opportunities for reminiscence about past child rearing experiences and
- provide tactile/sensory experiences that elicit a sense of comfort and security. (Dementia Behaviour Management Advisory Service, Victoria, 2009)

Contraindications and precautions

Assessment of the person with dementia's individual response needs to be handled with care and sensitivity. Not everyone will respond positively to the dolls, and it may even take some time to find one that elicits a therapeutic response. Be aware of staff or others who disregard this therapy as having therapeutic benefits – their negative responses may potentially affect the person with dementia's response. Consultation and education of staff and family can be facilitated by sharing guidelines and viewing the DVD 'Jack' (Alzheimer's Australia Tasmania, 2006). See Guidelines in Appendix 7.2 to assist with the introduction of the therapy.

Case study

Margaret was a 78-year-old lady living in a residential care home. Staff had referred her to the local Residential Support Program because of her increasing resistiveness to personal care and worsening verbal and physical aggression. Margaret had been a loving mother of four children, and parenting had been a very important part of her life. Following education of and consultation with Margaret's family and the staff, Doll Therapy was introduced. Not only did her signs of aggression settle, but she became more animated and conversant, and the doll satisfied her unmet need to care for others and provided meaning and purpose in her life. The family noted that once the doll was introduced, 'Mum became more involved in life and happier than we'd seen her for many months.' She took the doll with her when transferred to another facility, and it was an important source of continuity which was credited with helping her to make a smooth adjustment to her new environment.

Practical guidance and directions

To practice Complementary Therapies in this field, one can work in a number of ways:

1. Independently in one's own practice (if fully qualified),
2. Undertaking the therapy in an organization as a visiting professional (see Appendix 7.3),
3. Incorporating a therapy that one is qualified to practice, as part of another professional role (e.g. nurse) – this entails having the permission of one's employer and/or,
4. as part of the activities and therapies on offer to an organization's clientele (see Table 7.1 'Most suitable therapies for unqualified care staff', below).

From many years of direct experience and of also assisting others, the following '**7 Keys to Success**' are designed to assist with the practical application of Complementary Therapies in dementia care settings:

1. Don't go it alone
   a. Form a representative committee or working party with active members.
   b. Involve key stakeholders including people who have influence within the organization, as well as consumer representatives.
   c. Meet no more than bimonthly.
2. Start simply
   a. Set clear, achievable objectives.
   b. Establish a 'terms of reference'.
   c. Avoid the 'paradigm challenging' Complementary Therapies in the beginning.
3. Indentify potential barriers
   a. Be sensitive to language, culture and prejudice.
   b. Be aware of those who may seek to undermine or sabotage your efforts.
   c. Politically, target those who are most likely to be your detractors, and work hard to engage them.
   d. Do a cost–benefit analysis.

4. Do your homework!
   a. Consider and explore the following:
      i. Policies and procedures including Occupational Health and Safety,
      ii. Legal and ethical issues,
      iii. Practical issues including qualifications, external practitioners, storage of supplies and funding,
      iv. Quality issues (e.g. products used),
      v. Education of staff and information provided to carers,
      vi. Research opportunities.
5. Evaluate outcomes
   a. Ensure documentation and report back via Quality Improvement mechanisms including
      i. care Plan Reviews with family, doctor and
      ii. satisfaction surveys.
   b. Record changes in (e.g.)
      i. sleep/settling patterns,
      ii. behaviours of concern,
      iii. medication usage,
      iv. skin condition,
      v. budget.
6. Promote your activities
   a. Get some publicity including media, academic publications.
   b. Promote benefits for residents/patients, staff, families and the organization.
7. Don't give up!
   a. There ARE people out there that are on the same planet!
   b. Remember – *'It only takes one flea to irritate an entire dog!'* (Anon.)

Training requirements

It is advisable for staff to have some form of qualification if applying a particular therapy in the workplace, or at the very least, a qualified and experienced professional working alongside the carers in a consultancy capacity. There are a number of therapies that can be safely applied with minimal training, but background research and professional advice and input is important and advisable.

Table 7.1 Most suitable therapies for health and aged care workers who are not fully qualified in Complementary Therapies

Environmental manipulation	Music	Simple hand & Foot massage
Hug therapy	Simple guided imagery	Humour
Simple aromatherapy	Pet therapy	Child representational (doll) therapy

A cautionary reminder – KNOW YOUR CLIENT, DO YOUR HOMEWORK, INFORM & INVOLVE THE CARE TEAM & FAMILY, DOCUMENT ACTIVITIES & OUTCOMES.

If one decides to undertake a course in Complementary Therapies, the following questions may be helpful to consider:

- Is the course comprehensive or an overview? Is an introductory short course available that counts towards a qualification, so that the student has an opportunity to 'try' the therapy/course out before making the commitment to undertaking a longer course?
- Is it run by a recognized education institution that has achieved some external accreditation and/or is recognized by a relevant professional organization or association?
- Does completion of the course enable you to qualify for membership/registration with a recognized professional body and eligible for professional indemnity insurance?
- Is the course conducted at or through an education institution that has facilities that you require? – for example, library, study resources, well- equipped classrooms, access to child care, ongoing support once you've qualified and so on.
- If the course is conducted primarily 'online', how is the practical component of the training undertaken, and is it competency-based? Will you be given assistance in finding suitable practical experience opportunities to consolidate your training and practice?
- Are you able to get a total or partial refund should you withdraw from the course?

- Is there any recognition of prior relevant learning that may help with 'credits' towards subjects that you may have previously studied?
- It is often helpful to speak with past graduates of the institution, and to check with government agencies that the institution is registered and well-regarded.

Conclusions and the way forward

The reasons that Complementary Therapies are a popular and viable choice for the care of people with dementia are

- Complementary Therapies have been demonstrated to add quality to the lives of people with dementia;
- The non-invasiveness and gentle, even pleasant nature of many therapies comparative to modern Western medical practices;
- Although conventional treatments such as medications can delay and alleviate some symptoms, they all have side effects that can impact negatively on the health and well-being of the person with dementia; and
- Latest research indicates that non-pharmacological treatments are the most effective way to minimize and manage behavioural and psychological symptoms of dementia (Ames, 2009; Howard, 2008), and a number of Complementary Therapies lend themselves to this purpose;
- Complementary Therapies are also valuable as part of a palliative approach to dementia, from early to later and terminal stages. (Alzheimer's Australia, 2007; Australian Government NHMRC, 2006; Australian Pain Society, 2005)

This chapter has clearly illustrated how by their very nature Complementary Therapies can address each of Kitwood's person-centred needs. Just as importantly, however, is the fact that by undertaking these therapies as interventions, carers stand to benefit also, thus keeping them emotionally and spiritually nurtured as carers.

More research would certainly be helpful in continuing to provide evidence of the enormous benefits that Complementary

Therapies can bring to the care of people with dementia and their carers.

If Complementary Therapies are to be seen as legitimate interventions in the professional carer skill repertoire, they need to be offered formally as part of a competency-based carer curriculum. This will ensure that minimum knowledge, skill and practice standards are met. Likewise, health and aged care providers also need to meet their consumer's demands and cultivate a professional stance by having policies, procedures and quality improvement guidelines regarding Complementary Therapies. Unfortunately, if they continue as popular options that people often 'dabble' rather than formally train in, they run the risk of being used inappropriately. Critics and those suspicious of the merits of Complementary Therapies have been known to place blanket bans on the use of these therapies where instances of adverse reactions have occurred, and if such instances are not heeded, much of the good work undertaken, can unravel all too easily.

In conclusion, Complementary Therapies will succeed if they are implemented with considered preparation, planning and commitment. They can be effective and rewarding keys to a truly person-centred and holistic approach to dementia care with benefits for all involved.

> Death is not the ultimate tragedy of life. The ultimate tragedy is depersonalisation – dying (or living) in an alien and sterile area, separated from the spiritual nourishment that comes from being able to reach out to a loving hand, separated from a desire to experience things that make life worth living, separated from hope. (Cousins, 1979)

Appendix 7.1 – Aromatherapy washcloth procedure

Rationale

To provide guidelines for the safe and effective provision of aromatherapy wash cloths.

Indications

To promote a pleasant environment through the use of mood stabilizing essential oils, and to facilitate the washing of face and hands prior to meals, thereby reducing infection risk. To create a ritual for residents with dementia which helps to stimulate memory in regard to the serving of each meal (promoting food intake).

Table 7A.1   Standard operating procedure

Stage	Responsibility	Description
1	Care staff	**Assessment** **Discuss** the appropriateness of Aromatherapy Wash Cloth Procedure with the Unit Manager/ Residential Aged Care Manager. **Consult** with the patient/resident or their family/ representative about the possibility of therapy, the rationale for therapy, the associated costs and any possible side effects. Document verbal consent in the progress notes. **Check** for contraindications and precautions, including allergy to essential oils.
2.	Care Staff	**Equipment** Glass bowl Face washers Warm water Disposable gloves Tongs Plastic bags (1 for every 10 washers) **Essential Oils**: Ensure that only organization-approved essential oils are used.
3.	Care Staff	**Procedure** Half fill bowl with warm tap water. Place maximum total of 10 drops of essential oils per litre of water. Wash and dry hands thoroughly, prior to glove application. Wearing gloves, gently agitate the water to mix through the oils, and then add no more than 10 of the face washers at a time (folded into quarters) to the water. Squeeze out excess water from washers, and place in one of the plastic bags. Repeat process for remaining washers, placing them in another plastic bag. Place in microwave oven for 40 seconds on high. Using tongs, hand out washers to each resident one table at a time, gently shaking out the washer to reduce excess steam and heat. Supervise and prompt as required with face and hand cleaning, collect used washers, place in laundry receptacle. Clean bowl following use with hot soapy water.

Appendix 7.2 – Guidelines for Doll Therapy

- Greet the person as you enter their room, cradling the doll in your arms (you may like to have it wrapped in a small blanket), and then sit down with them.
- Observe how the person responds to the doll in your arms. If they have not noticed it, bring the doll to their attention and invite their feedback. If the person appears interested and engaged, invite them to hold it.
- Make general comments about the doll (e.g. 'his/her' appearance), taking care not to identify it as either a doll or baby at this stage.
- Observe how the person interacts with the doll and whether they appear to be identifying it as a real baby.
- Mirror the person's response, that is, only act as if it is a real baby if the person themselves appear to exhibit that belief.
- Ask if they would like to look after the baby whilst you attend to other duties, reassuring them that you will return.
- Leave a bassinette/capsule/basket in reach and reassure the person that they can place it in this if they get tired.
- Place the doll in a bassinette/capsule/basket near the person when not in use to enable the person to pick up the doll at will and as the opportunity arises.
- Monitor and evaluate the success of the intervention in providing the person with pleasure, and meaningful activity.
- Determine the best times to use this form of therapy according to the individual's needs. At times it will be necessary to remove the doll from the person, that is, for meal times/showering and so on. This will need to be done sensitively as some individuals may be extremely protective and defensive in their reactions. Offering to put the doll 'down for a nap', 'feed' it or 'change its nappy' may be used as logical reasons for why you are taking it away. Reassure the person that you will bring the doll back (and follow through with this commitment).
- (Adapted from St Vincent's Aged Psychiatry Service, 2007)

Appendix 7.3 – Framework for a professional procedural template *to engage Complementary Therapists* (not directly employed by the organization such as a nursing home or hospital)

Procedure: 'Complementary Therapies – authorization for therapists to practice'

Rationale: Therapists not employed directly by the organization may apply for authorization to practice on site.

Stage	Responsibility	Description
1		**Application process.** Complete documentation including personal contact details, qualifications, membership of a recognized professional association, relevant work history, professional development activity and proof of indemnity and liability insurance and a recent police check.
2		**Assess application.** Arrange for interview and check referees. Process through HR as per external contractor policy.
3		**Payment arrangements and fees.** Client or their representative may be invoiced directly by practitioner; however, in residential care the client's Trust account may be invoiced.
4		**Equipment and supplies.** Practitioner is responsible for supply and maintenance of equipment and consumables. Any electrical equipment is to be checked and tagged by the facility's engineering service. All equipment is to be in good working order and compliant with safety standards and regulations.
5		**Informed consent.** Verbal consent is obtained from the client or their representative prior to commencement of Complementary Therapies, following an explanation of the therapy and proposed treatment plan. Documented in client's records.
6		**Privacy and security.** Therapist is to prearrange visits, report arrival and departure to person in charge of facility at the time. Arrangements are made to ensure quiet, secure and private service location with appropriate signage on display.

Stage	Responsibility	Description
7		**Documentation of therapy.** Documentation of assessment, treatment and outcome is required, and the authorized practitioner is permitted to access client records for this purpose. Any concerns or queries that the practitioner may have regarding the client are to be directed to the person in charge.
8		**Incident reporting.** Any untoward event is to be reported to the person in charge immediately and an incident form completed.
9		**Adherence to organization policies and regulations.** Authorized practitioners agree to adhere to policies including Occupational Health and Safety, Privacy and Confidentiality and so on, as discussed at interview and provided at orientation.

References

Access Economics (April) (2009). Making choices. Future dementia care: projections, problems and preferences. Report by Access Economics Pty Limited for Alzheimer's Australia. www.alzheimers.org.au, accessed 9 Jan 2011.

Alzheimer's Australia (2007). *Quality Dementia Care Standards: A Guide to Practice for Managers.* www.alzheimers.org.au/upload/QDC21.pdf, accessed 14 March 2010.

Alzheimer's Australia (2009). *Dementia Care Essentials Training Program.* NSW, Australia: Alzheimer's Australia Victoria.

Alzheimer's Australia (2008). *New Housing and Renovations: The Environment and Dementia (Help Sheet)* www.alzheimers.org.au, accessed 14 March 2010.

Alzheimer's Australia Tasmania (2006). www.alzheimers.org.au/Tasmania.

Alzheimer's Society UK (2009) Fact sheet no 434: complementary and alternative medicines and dementia. See alzheimers.org.uk, accessed 9/1/2011.

Ames, Prof. D. (2009). Changed Behaviours in older people with cognitive impairment – why they matter. Presentation at Change Champions 'Managing Challenging Behaviours' conference, Melbourne Victoria, May 2009.

Australian Government (2008). *Dementia Resource Guide.* www.health.gov.au/dementia, accessed 14 March 2010.

Australian Government National Health & Medical Research Council (2006). *Guidelines for Palliative Approach in Residential*

Aged Care. www.nhmrc.gov.au/synopses/ac12to14syn.htm, accessed 9 Jan 2011.

Australian Pain Society (2005). *Improving Management of Pain in Aged Care Facilities.* http://www.health.gov.au/internet/ministers/publishing.nsf/Content/health-mediarel-yr2005-jb-bis154.htm.

Ballard, C. G., O'Brien, J. T., Reichelt, K. & Perry, E. K. (2002). Aromatherapy as a safe and effective treatment for the management of agitation in severe dementia: the results of a double blind, placebo-controlled trial of Melissa. *Journal of Clinical Psychiatry,* July 63(7), 553–558.

Benson, H. & Klipper, M. Z. (1977). *The Relaxation Response.* London: Collins.

Bird, M. (2009). A case specific approach to challenging behaviour associated with dementia. Presentation at Change Champions 'Managing Challenging Behaviour' conference, Melbourne, Victoria, Australia May 2009.

Burns, G. (1996). Memories of abuse: fact or fiction? Presentation at the Mind Body Connection Conference, Gawler Foundation. 8–11 March, Lorne, Victoria, Australia.

Bush, E. (2001). The Use of human touch to improve the well-being of older adults. *J Holist Nurs* Vik 19, no 3, 256–270.

Commonwealth Respite and Carelink Centre, Southern Region (2009). Creative Ways to Care – Strategies for carers of people living with dementia. Caulfield Hospital (A member of Alfred Health). www.carersouth.org.au, accessed 13 April 2010.

Cousins, N. (1979). *Anatomy of an Illness As Perceived by the Patient: Reflections on Healing and Regeneration.* New York: Norton.

Dementia Behaviour Management Advisory Service, Victoria (2009). *Guidelines for Child Representational (Doll) Therapy and Pet Therapy (2010).* Melbourne: St Vincent's Hospital. Can be obtained from dbmas@svhm.org.au

Dunning, T. (ed.) (2006). *Complementary Therapies and the Management of Diabetes and Vascular Disease – A Matter of Balance.* Chichester, West Sussex, England: John Wiley & Sons Ltd.

Dunning, T. (2007). *Essential Oils in Therapeutic Care.* Melbourne, Victoria: Australian Scholarly Publishing.

Ebersole, P., Hess, P. A. & Schmidt Luggen, A. (2004). *Toward Healthy Aging: Human Needs and Nursing Response* (7th Ed.). St Louis, MO Elsevier

Gurvich, T. & Cunningham, J. A. (2000). Appropriate use of psychotropic drugs in nursing homes. *American Family Physician,* 61, 1437–1446.

Holmes, C., Hopkins, V., Hensford, C., Mac Laughlin, V., Wilkinson, D. & Rosenvinge, H. (2001). Lavender oil as a treatment for agitated behaviour in severe dementia – a placebo controlled trial. *International Journal of Geriatric Psychiatry*, 17, 305–308.

Howard, Prof. R. (2008). Address to Ageing and Mental Health Annual Scientific Meeting, Melbourne University, 27–28 November 2008.

Innes, A. & Hatfield, K. (eds) (2001). *Healing Art Therapies and Person-Centred Dementia Care*. London: Jessica Kingsley Publishers.

James, K. (2006). Thesis: *An anchor in chaotic seas – staff perceptions of the impact of a systematic meal protocol on residents in a dementia-specific nursing unit*. St. Albans (Melbourne) Victoria: Victoria University.

Joanna Briggs Institute (2008). The JBI Approach to Evidence-Based Practice (Levels of evidence). www.joannabriggs.edu.au, Accessed 9/1/11.

Manheimer, E. & Berman, B. (2007). Cochrane Complementary Medicine Field: Scope and topics.

McCabe, P. (ed.) (2001). *Complementary Therapies in Nursing and Midwifery – From Vision to Practice*. Ascot Vale (Melbourne): Ausmed Publications.

Memory Bridge (Chicago, USA). www.memorybridge.org, videos – Gladys Wilson.

Moyle, Prof. W. (2008). Complementary therapies: do they have a role in the treatment of disruptive behaviours? Presentation delivered 27 February 2008 at University of Wollongong, NSW for Eastern Australia Dementia Training & Study Centre.

National Institute of Complementary Medicine (NICM) (2009). Australia www.nicm.edu.au, accessed 9 Jan 2011.

Nurses Board of Victoria (1999). *Guidelines for Complementary Therapies*. Melbourne, Victoria, Australia: NBV.

O'Connor, D., Ames, D., Gardner, B. & King, M. (2009). Psychosocial treatments of behavioural symptoms in dementia: a systematic review of reports. *International Psychogeriatrics*, 21, 225–240.

Olsen, K. (1992). *The Encyclopaedia of Alternative Health Care – The Complete Guide of Choices in Healing*. London: Judy Piatkus Publishers.

Pert, C. (1997). *Molecules of Emotion: Why You Feel the Way You Feel*. New York: Scribner.

Rankin-Box, D. (ed.) (1995). *The Nurses' Handbook of Complementary Therapies*. Edinburgh: Churchill Livingstone.

Schneider, S. L., Tariot, P. N., Dagerman, K. S. et al. (2006). Effectiveness of atypical antipsychotic drugs in patients with Alzheimer's disease. *The New England Journal of Medicine*, 355, 1525–1538 12 October 2006, No 15.

Sierpina, V. S., Sierpina, M., Loera, J. A. & Grumbles, L. (2005). Complementary and integrative approaches to dementia: mind-body therapies. *Southern Medical Journal*, 98(6), 636–645.

State Government of Victoria (2009). Better Health Channel Complementary Therapies Fact Sheet www.betterhealth.vic.gov.au, accessed 19 April 2010.

St Vincent's Aged Psychiatry (2007). *Residential Support Program. Doll Therapy Brochure.* Kew, Victoria, Australia: St Vincent's Health, c/- St. George's Hospital.

Taylor, B. (2001). "Research Issues in Complementary Therapies and Holistic Care" in McCabe P (ed.) *Complementary Therapies in Nursing and Midwifery – From Vision to Practice.* Ascot Vale (Melbourne): Ausmed Publications.

Trout, S. (1990). *To See Differently – Personal Growth and Being of Service Through Attitudinal Healing.* Washington, DC: Three Roses Press.

Vickers, A. (1996). *Massage and Aromatherapy – A Guide for Health Professionals.* London: Chapman & Hall.

Zimmerman, S., Williams, C. S., Reed, P. S., Boustani, M., Priesser, J. S., Heck, E., Sloan, P. D. (2005). Attitudes, stress and satisfaction of staff who care for residents with dementia. *The Gerontologist,* 45(Special Issue 1), 96–105.

Further Reading

Brett, H. (2002). *Complementary Therapies in the Care of Older People.* London: Whurr Publishing.

Freeman, L. W. & Lawlis, F. G. (2001). *Mosby's Complementary & Alternative Medicine – A Research-based Approach.* Missouri: Mosby Inc.

Graham, H. (1999). *Complementary Therapies in Context – The Psychology of Healing.* London: Jessica Kingsley Publishers.

Mackenzie, E. & Rakel, B. (2006). *Complementary & Alternative Medicine for Older Adults: A Guide to Holistic Approaches to Healthy Ageing.* New York: Springer Publishing Co Inc.

Rankin-Box, D. (ed.) (2001). *The Nurse's Handbook of Complementary Therapies* (2nd Ed.). London: Bailliere Tindall.

Spencer, J. W. & Jacobs, J. J. (eds) (1999). *Complementary/Alternative Medicine – An Evidence-based Approach.* Missouri: Mosby Inc.

Waring, L. A. (2000). *Assessment for Reaching People with Dementia Through Their Senses.* Scotland: Dementia Services Development Centre, University of Stirling (useful document outlining assessments pre and post therapeutic interventions)

Weir, M. (2000). *Complementary Medicine: Ethics and Law.* Brisbane: Prometheus Publications.

www.health.vic.gov.au/dpu/resource-kit.htm, accessed 19 April 2010 (due to be revised 2010) – (letters and policy frameworks to assist implementation of Complementary Therapies).

8 Story matters in dementia care

Trisha Kotai-Ewers

Irene, a resident in a dementia hostel whose words the author recorded over a long period of time.

Introduction

Case study

I first met Evie when she moved into the hostel where I worked as a writer recording the words of people with dementia. She was standing in the lounge room, arms hugged closely around her chest, head bent. Her eyes stared vacantly. I touched her gently on the arm. 'You look lost.' 'I've been lost ever since I came here.' With that, she retreated into silence and further conversation was impossible.

Later in the afternoon a carer led her outside to join a group of us sitting in the sun. I was not recording any words at the time. Perhaps it was the warmth of the sun, perhaps the relaxed atmosphere. No matter what caused it, Evie opened up and started to talk about the way memories came. With gentle prompting by a carer, she spoke of her family. Everyone joined in the general sharing of stories, which continued in an animated way for almost an hour and a quarter, with Evie as principal narrator.

After this exhilarating exchange of stories, the group broke up and Evie disappeared indoors. Ten minutes later she emerged to stand before us, flung her arms wide and laughingly exclaimed, 'Here's the storyteller back again!' It was wonderful to see the transformation. Her body language said it all. With that simple act of telling her recollections of childhood to a group of sympathetic listeners, she had transformed from a withdrawn, lost being to an expansive, smiling woman. And she had remembered the activity of a short time ago (Kotai-Ewers, 2007).

We all enjoy sharing our stories and having them heard by those around us. Whether it is what happened on our way to work that morning, our holiday adventures or childhood memories, we relate to other people through our stories. Even more important, however, as psychologists acknowledge, we need to tell our stories to maintain a sense of our own identity. Telling our stories helps us make sense of our present and our past, and to understand who we are (McAdams et al., 2006). This is true for everyone, no matter their age or circumstance. Nores (1997) in a Finnish study to identify which elements of their care were most important to older people living in residential care settings found results which might surprise some care providers. The residents in the study listed elements such as 'participating in sufficient daily activities' or 'receiving gentle care' as being of lesser importance to their well-being. At the top of the list they placed factors such as 'being understood', 'being heard' and 'being able to be one's self'. The older people who participated in this study, none of whom had dementia, wanted above all to be able to tell their stories and to know that these stories were heard and accepted as valid. It is likely, however, that people with dementia have a far greater need to tell their stories and have them heard and accepted. Given the many losses they undergo with the onset of memory loss and the lack of what seems to be any real future ahead for them, their stories may provide a potent strategy to avert depression and anxiety. The stories may also be seen as counteracting some of the twofold stigma of age and mental illness which our society so often attaches to the elderly with dementia (Crisp, 1995, 1999).

When John Killick moved from recording the life histories of frail residents in old people's homes to the role of writer in residence with people with dementia, he chose to immerse himself in their daily life by living with them in a dementia-specific residence for the first week. Writing of this experience John described how, after feeling most uncomfortable and even threatened for the first 48 hours in the unit, everything changed for him when the other residents began to approach him and share their thoughts and feelings with him. As soon as communication was established two things happened. John lost his apprehension of the residents and they 'suddenly became people' for him. Hearing their stories had created a sense of fellow humanity and empathy. The residents in that dementia-specific care unit certainly wanted to tell their stories. They were the ones who sought John out and initiated the communication (Killick & Allan, 2001).

Evidence base

When, in 1997, I became a writer working with people with dementia in Perth, Western Australia, I used John's booklet *Please Give Me Back My Personality!* (Killick, 1994) as my guide. I was also supported by grief-counsellor and psychotherapist Judy Griffiths. Thanks to initial funding from Alzheimer's Australia, we met fortnightly over several years to discuss and elucidate the words as I recorded them. As a child, I had watched my mother care for her father during the seven years that he lived with us before his death at the age of 93. As an adult, I was my mother's principal carer until her death at the age of 94. This latter experience led me to this work of listening to and recording the stories of people with dementia.

Like John, in order to record the words of people at different stages of dementia, I worked in residential care units as well as day care centres. Over many years I recorded thousands of words, sometimes following one person from the relatively early stages of dementia until their move into full-time care and ultimate loss of language. At other times I might see someone only once or twice. No matter who they were, or at what stage of the disease, they expressed appreciation at being able to speak freely and having their words accepted. As Ces said, 'You help some ...' 'Me?''Yes, you.' 'Does it help?' .... 'Oh, yes!' (Kotai-Ewers, 2007). From someone with very little ability to communicate in words, this last response was uttered with great emphasis and a surprising sureness.

During this time, people with dementia spoke to me about a wide variety of subjects including their family and friends, their care, death and attempts to find meaning. Most frequently, however, they wanted to tell me about the experience of having dementia. While very few could still name the problem, they all knew that they were somehow different from their earlier self. May, a regular visitor to a day care centre, spoke in some detail of her feelings about these changes:

> I don't like what I am now...My back's gone...my leg's gone...My head's gone...It is quite a lot to think about. There's lots of things I don't talk about because I can't remember. Now I can't do anything. I've got no way. I've never had it before. I've got to wait and see which way it goes.

Case study

May painted a clear picture of the losses in her life. Some were physical, others emotional, like loss of direction and purpose. She was obviously searching for meaning now that her life has changed so dramatically. Her words showed an awareness of the effect of dementia upon her memory and the insecurity these losses caused.

Case study

Marjorie, with whom I had many conversations over several years, taught me more of the losses experienced by people with dementia. Early on, she expressed a lot of anger about living in a dementia hostel when she said, 'I am really very angry ... I have a right to a life of my own ... I just want to be at home and be myself.' I found those last two words most significant. Whereas Marjorie had no name for what was happening to her, she, like May, knew that she did not feel 'herself'. Over time, I explored what Marjorie meant by the word 'home'. Sometimes it was England, the land of her birth. At other times it was the apartment she lived in before moving into the hostel. I learned a lot about her earlier life. An only child, whose father was killed during the war, Marjorie had developed a close relationship with her mother. Alone after two failed marriages, Marjorie lived in Perth while her only son lived in England. Being alone was an essential part of her life. Now, however, she lived with 15 other people, as well as the carers. She even shared a room with another woman. Marjorie had no opportunity for the solitude that had no doubt become necessary for her in order to feel herself. For some time while I was recording her words, her room-mate spent weeks in hospital before moving to another facility. During that time Marjorie had the room to herself and could retreat from the noise and 'busy-ness' of the hostel. One day, however, I arrived to find a carer pounding on the locked door of her room. A new resident was now sharing the room and Marjorie was making her own protest by locking her out. Being aware of her preference for solitude, reinforced by years of living alone, I could only sympathize. Marjorie was responding in the only way she could to the losses suffered by a solitary person moving into hostel care. I wonder how many people like Marjorie are living in communal settings which are quite foreign to their personal preferences (Kotai-Ewers, 2007).

Case study

Often the stories told by people with dementia resemble the disjointed nature of a dream. Knowing something of their earlier life can help us unravel the threads in the same way that it helped me understand Marjorie's actions. In my few conversations with Rae, I was at first confused by the stories she wove involving a violinist, the Catholic Church and playing the violin for the Pope in Rome. To my uninformed mind, it all seemed a complicated figment of her imagination. However, when I spoke to her sister I learned that an uncle had been a gifted violinist, performing in concert halls around the world until he became a Catholic priest. Rae was sharing with me part of her family history. When my mother moved from the dementia hostel to nursing home care, I learned more of the value of supplying life histories for people with dementia. As requested by the staff, I supplied a brief account of her life. Reading it, a senior nurse realized that my father had taught her mother in a small country school in the mid-1920s. This connection, and the fact that he had been a very popular teacher, ensured that my mother always retained her individuality. That nurse helped me bathe my mother's body after her death.

Rae spoke repeatedly about being 'in the dark'. In the middle of her other complex stories she would return to the same theme. When she had a psychotic episode, she pulled down the curtains from her windows. Perhaps she was not being merely destructive but wanted to let the light into her darkness.

Case study

Irene also vented her rage on the curtains in moments of instability, often unpicking the seams. Over many long conversations she had told me of her life 'in the old times' growing up on a farm where she helped her father, who 'was the bushy around the town'. She also helped her mother in the house with the 'lots of sisters'. Irene was never sure how many sisters there were. I wondered how someone as active as she had been could adjust to the inactivity of residential care. Did she unpick the curtains in an attempt to counteract the apparent lack of purpose in her present life? If so, what implications does this have for institutionalized aged care? Is there some way that we can adjust our practices in order to help residents retain a sense of meaning in their lives and to allow for the individual differences they have developed over their long lifetime?

Good practice

Case study

I saw the success of such adaptations when I worked with Grant for some years. At the age of 49, he was quite out of place in a day care centre among the other daily visitors whose average age was probably between 75 and 80. As a gourmet cook and wine connoisseur, he found little in the daily activities to encourage him to return each week. Before the onset of Alzheimer's disease he had lectured in Occupational Therapy at a local university. Staff used this information to make special arrangements for Grant, giving him access to staff conversations, letting him bring his own lunch and usually spend the day with just one carer rather than mix with the other visitors. For many months I spent Wednesdays with Grant, talking in a quiet room or outside in the garden, where his language became noticeably more fluent. Some days we walked in nearby bushland or went to a café for coffee. I also visited him in respite homes and when he finally moved into full-time care. No matter where we met he retained an awareness of me as a writer and an interest in what I was writing, with comments like

> Write bits and pieces – funny things if you can – there's funny things like cabbages and things – Look around for things. We can talk a lot – Mostly I'm very sensible.

Like many people in the early stages of dementia, Grant at first tried to keep a journal so that his friends and family would know how he felt. He commented acerbically on the treatment he received from doctors and health professionals in the early days, saying that his social worker wife could

> talk to doctors in psychologese, but the strange thing is that they talk to her about my ailments with her rather than me. When this happens, and it happens regularly, I feel like a child whose ailments are discussed by grown-ups with hardly any reference to the body in question who is too young to know what is really going on. At best it's demeaning to the patient and at worst it's insulting to anyone whose mind is still functioning quite well in most areas necessary for a normal life. Having taught courses to students in Physiotherapy and Occupational Therapy for some years I feel insulted by those who assume that I have very little to contribute to discussions on my condition.

> The last time I saw him Grant could no longer speak, but all the same, he communicated in a way that gave me a most valuable insight. I told him I would not be visiting him anymore because I had to concentrate on writing the book about my work. He stretched his arms out in front of him and moved his fingers as if he were typing on a keyboard. He had heard and understood my words and was agreeing that now was the time for me to write.

Over the years I became convinced that people with dementia understood most of what I said to them, and that their stories invariably contained kernels of fact. I also became aware that these facts held major significance for the storyteller.

I was continuously struck by the similarity of these accounts to dreams, where elements of past and present intermingle, against apparently fantastic backgrounds. Jungian psychologists work almost exclusively with their clients' dreams. Should the dream be recurring it is seen as having special meaning for the dreamer. Can we apply this to the often-repeated stories of people with dementia?

Case study

While encouraging a group of people in a nursing home to tell their stories, Ffranses Ingram was struck by one resident's repeated story. Over and over he spoke of a shipwreck off the coast of Wales 70 years before, which left all the crew except himself either dead or injured. He expressed deep guilt at the fact that he was the only sailor who escaped without harm. Acting on his information, Ffranses contacted the priest in the village where most of the crew grew up. He verified the story, sending back to the nursing home photos and stories of the men and their families. He also put flowers on the graves of those who died. This verification of his story and the act of recognition for those who died appeared to relieve some of the guilt the man had carried all those years (Ingram, 1997).

As a writer in residence I was able to simply be with people, allow them to talk when and as they chose, without any of the other responsibilities of staff for the day-to-day business of the facilities. It is much harder for carers with the responsibility for attending to people's physical needs to feel able to take this time and give this concentrated attention, although, it is possible more often than we believe. One carer, concerned at the depth of sorrow a resident was expressing, took the opportunity to set time aside and really listen to the woman's words. She shared them with me later. At first it had been hard to make any sense out of the jumble of past and present, peppered with the names of family members. Gradually a theme emerged. The speaker felt sad for all 'those poor things who didn't want to stay' and for the others who 'got lost inside the house and had to be shown where to go'. This was particularly revealing to the carer as the resident seemed inclined to be a loner who did not like group activities or communicating with other residents. It appeared she had a much deeper empathy with her fellow residents than had been imagined. She was also telling the carer how very unhappy she was at being in the hostel. People with dementia frequently speak in metaphors. Very often conversations apparently about other people in reality refer to the speaker. So, in this case, the 'poor things who didn't want to stay' also referred to the resident herself. Some carers might feel uncomfortable to know such feelings, but it is essential for any understanding of and communication with people in care (Cheston, 1996). Only when we can empathize with people can we really meet their needs.

Over the past 15 years there have been many exciting developments that endorse communication with people with dementia. Australian linguist Jane Crisp began listening to her mother's stories with the attentive and open mind of someone fascinated by language and its uses (Crisp, 1995, 1999 & 2000). Her articles and book encourage us to enjoy the fact that people with dementia still want to share their stories with us. An increasing number of individual programs and events throughout the world are based on providing the possibility of sharing stories in the dementia care setting, from employing storytellers or writers to intergenerational projects where students meet elders with dementia and hear their stories. Innovative programs have sprung up in the public domain as well. In the United States, museums and art galleries like the Museum of Fine Arts in Boston and the Museum of Modern Art in New York run special programs which facilitate visits and discussions by people with dementia as they respond to the artworks.

Increasingly we hear the voice of people with dementia either through publications like retired psychologist Dr Richard Taylor's 'Alzheimer's from the Inside Out' (Taylor, 2006), through public talks and conferences. Since the early 2000s, conferences have increasingly included a stream presented by people with a recent diagnosis of dementia. In 2008, Toronto in Canada hosted a conference organized and presented entirely by people with dementia and their carers. Richard Taylor was one of the speakers and wrote that it was 'amazingly wonderful to be there' (Taylor, 2008). Such events, though isolated, form part of a stream of opportunities now available especially to people in the early stages of the condition, to tell their stories to the general population and more especially to carers. Recent discoveries of brain plasticity which show that our brains can adapt to changes in structure and develop new pathways for transferring information have also suggested new hope that by keeping our brains active and working in new ways, we may be able to retain healthy thought processes further into old age than was ever dreamed possible (Doidge, 2007).

Some of the new alternatives, based on person-centred care, which have become popular in recent years, are fully discussed elsewhere in this book. One which has been wide-spread since its inception in the United States in 1991 is the Eden Alternative. Reacting against what they saw as a model of departmentalized and task-oriented institutional facilities, Dr William Thomas and his wife developed a model which aims to include care for the human spirit as well as the body, which tends to be the focus in the majority of establishments (Thomas, 1996). There are now over 300 registered homes, in the United States, Canada, Europe and Australia, and while the original concept applied to the care of older people in general, Eden Alternative in Australia has successfully used the vision to transform dementia care in some day care centres in particular. By creating more homely settings where children, pets and plants are welcome, the Eden Alternative hopes to create meaningful care centres which will go a long way towards eliminating the loneliness, helplessness and boredom which are all too often present in everyday dementia care.

All of these activities, however, are what I would call 'from the top down'. Their implementation usually requires major support from governing bodies through organization and often specific funding. Everyday carers of people with dementia, whether in day centres or residential homes, can feel isolated from such measures. Yet real heart-to-heart communication is probably most effective when it takes place within the care unit in the most natural way possible. The story of Evie with which I began this chapter is a perfect example of such a natural storytelling episode, which lightened the spirits of both the storyteller and her listeners. It is possible for carers to communicate at a deeper level with people with dementia within the framework of daily activities once there is a more general understanding of some very specific ways in which dementia affects a person's ability to communicate verbally.

Practical guidance

There are ten steps which can help us find our way through the often confusing labyrinth of story as told by people with dementia (Kotai-Ewers, 2007).

Opening the Door. For meaningful communication to take place the carer needs to recognize what powerful medicine telling one's story can be, and be prepared to make an effort to hear those stories. If we approach each person's story with the acceptance that they want to communicate, and indeed have something meaningful to say, it will be easier to find that meaning.

Listening with the heart. This is a process of acceptance, of refraining from judgement no matter what peculiarities of speech or mannerism are present. A judgemental approach helps us to keep people at a distance, rather than engage with someone at heart level. By listening with the heart, we not only connect with the speaker but we are enriched by that connection.

Being totally present. People only feel truly heard if the listener is really present to the speaker. So often we find it difficult to just be instead of doing. One day in a hostel for people with dementia, as I sat waiting for someone to come and speak with me, I took out my journal and began writing. No one came near me all afternoon. As I packed the journal away, Marjorie approached me saying, 'We didn't like to disturb you. We could see you were busy.' I had missed a whole afternoon of stories just because I felt uncomfortable sitting waiting! We need to learn not to fill the space up with unnecessary activity. Why not, instead of a game of dominoes or bingo, use a free moment for conversation, for listening with the heart?

Embracing the irrational. Our Western society is dominated by scientific thought and its insistence on the rational and logical. There can be a sense of release in abandoning this domination from time to time. Instead of concentrating on how disturbing we find the apparent irrationality of stories told by people with dementia, we need to look beyond the surface confusion. Irene's failure to remember how many sisters she had in no way detracted from the richness of her stories.

Playing with language. Enjoying the way people with dementia play with language is part of letting go of the rational. Irene had a wonderful vocabulary all her own. A handkerchief was a 'sniff-sniff', laughter was a 'guggle' and she called herself a 'slower'. She may have meant 'loner', have invented a new word or even have meant she was both 'slow' and a loner. If a woman with dementia refers to her family as 'friends', does it mean she has forgotten who they are or that her brain and tongue cannot locate the 'family' words? Thanks to this work, I have realized the degree to which our brains store words in meaning groups. Nouns expressing relationships can often be mixed up, but people aren't usually referred to as inanimate objects or animals. More important than naming things or people correctly is the underlying feeling that is expressed.

Groping through grammar. Confusions of grammar manifest as past/present replacements and problems with syntax. Pronouns are frequently confused so that 'he', 'she' and 'they' can all appear in the same sentence and refer to the same person. I also found some very literal interpretations. When the carers were wearing trousers, they invariably became 'he'.

Uncovering metaphor. Many researchers have realized that people with dementia often speak in metaphors. Concealed within apparent inaccuracies we find that language has been used figuratively and so conveys ever-deeper meanings to a careful listener. John Killick pointed out that 'the disinhibiting effect of the disease' effectively released an untapped ability to use language symbolically (Killick, 2005). I was always struck by Irene's metaphor for death, when she spoke of going 'up' (or sometimes 'down') a ladder. 'I wonder when it exists when we fall down the ladder?' and, 'But I know quite well I'm up the ladder …' These phrases recurred consistently as she pondered the meaning of life and death.

Enjoying the story. When we relax the rational mind's demand for exact words, correct structures and facts, when we relax into a conversation based on feeling and empathy, then we can simply enjoy the story we are being told and through our enjoyment we give enjoyment to the storyteller. This is the essence of true communication. There can be communication beyond words, as Grant showed me on the last time I saw him. There can be communication even with those who seem beyond communicating. One of the greatest gifts my mother received in the weeks just before her death was the time a young carer spent, sitting by her bedside reading the English translation of Antoine de St Exupéry's French classic, *The Little Prince*. It seemed a perfect preparation for death, and hearing is the sense that remains until the end.

Nor must we forget that there is a form of communication beyond words, through a look, a smile or the touch of a hand. Very often this is the only way left for us to communicate with people in the later stages of dementia, and yet it can be just as powerful, just as reassuring.

Facing the feelings. Marie Mills has shown that in spite of failures in mental capabilities, people with dementia still experience strong feelings (Mills, 1998). Stories are often our means of coping with our emotions. When Wendy told me that her mother and father were dead, she was not reliving the past, but letting me know that when we spoke she felt as sad and bereft as she had when they died. Their death was a metaphor for her present feelings. By hearing and acknowledging these feelings the listener offers a gift to the speaker.

Revealing the treasure. All labyrinths hold a treasure at their centre. Here there are gifts for both listener and speaker. Evie's story illustrates clearly the release available through telling our stories and having them accepted. Listening with the heart confirms the listener's own sense of their identity, and offers insight into another's life and emotions.

Way forward

I hope that the voice of people diagnosed with dementia will continue to be heard not only in the conference hall but also in print, and increasingly in the popular media like radio, television and the Internet. However my deepest hope is that everyone reading these pages will realize the extent to which they can make a difference, not only to the people with dementia for whom they care, but in their own lives, by opening up to a deeper level of communication. We don't need to wait for large movements, huge expense accounts or months of professional development before we can change the nature of dementia care. We do need the courage to be open and to listen with the heart and without judgement. We will be enriching our own lives when we realize the importance of telling one's story in any care situation, and take steps to make time for such storytelling. The healing power of stories lies in their ability to encourage social interaction, to recreate the order of past times and refute the stigmas associated with old age. In so doing they help to reconstruct the identity of the teller, an identity that is threatened by the very nature of dementia and the experience of institutionalized care. Accepting that people with dementia do have understanding and do have something valuable to tell us, and really listening to their words, are essential steps on the way towards ensuring that their care is truly person-centred.

References

Cheston, R. (1996). Stories and metaphor: talking about the past in a psychotherapy group for people with dementia. *Ageing and Society*, 16, 579–602.

Crisp, J. (1995). Making sense of stories that people with Alzheimer's tell: a journey with my mother. *Nursing Inquiry*, 2, 133–140.

Crisp, J. (1995). Dementia and Communication. In Garrett, S. and Hamilton-Smith, E. (eds), *Rethinking Dementia: an Australian approach*, Melbourne: Ausmed Publications.

Crisp, J. (2000). *Keeping in Touch with Someone Who Has Alzheimer's*. Ascot Vale, Victoria: Ausmed Publications.

Doidge, N. (2007). *The Brain that Changes Itself: Stories of Personal Triumph from the Frontiers of Brain Science*. Melbourne: Scribe Publications Pty, Ltd.

Ingram, F. (1997). Every nursing home needs a storyteller. *Geriaction*, 15(4), 29–31.

Killick, J. (1994). *Please Give Me Back My Personality!* Stirling: DSDC, University of Stirling.

Killick, J. (2005). Making sense of dementia through metaphor. *Journal of Dementia Care*, 13(1), 22–23.

Killick, J. & Allan, K. (2001). *Communication and the Care of People with Dementia.* Buckingham: Open University Press. pp. 12–14.

Kotai-Ewers, T. (2007). *Listen to the Talk of Us: People with Dementia Speak Out.* Perth, Western Australia: Alzheimer's Australia (WA).

McAdams, D. P., Josselson, R., Lieblich, A. (eds) (2006). *Identity and Story: Creating Self in Narrative.* Washington, DC: APA (American Psychological Association) Publications.

Mills, M. A. (1998). *Narrative Identity and Dementia: A study of autobiographical memories and emotions.* Aldershot, England: Ashgate Publishing Ltd.

Nores, T. H. (1997). What is most important for elders in institutional care in Finland? *Geriatric Nursing,* 18(2), 67–69.

Taylor, R. (2006). *Alzheimer's from the Inside Out.* Baltimore: Health Professionals Press, Inc.

Taylor, R. (2008). Newsletter *Alzheimer's from the Inside Out.* November 2008, Issue #9.

Thomas, W. M. D. (1996). *Life Worth Living: How Someone You Love Can Still Enjoy Life in a Nursing Home. the Eden Alternative in Action.* Acton, MA: VanderWyk & Burnham.

9 Innovative approaches to reminiscence: remembering yesterday, caring today

Pam Schweitzer

Introduction

This chapter will explore the development of reminiscence as a means of supporting people affected by dementia. I shall call on wide experience of work in care homes and in the community in the United Kingdom (UK) and other European countries to show how a growing body of knowledge and skill concerning reminiscence in dementia care has developed over the past 15 years.

This chapter demonstrates how the cross-fertilization of ideas and approaches from different, and apparently unconnected disciplines, has opened up opportunities for learning and development for people with dementia, their family carers and those who work with them in health, social care, medical and community fields. It suggests how the use of skills and the attitudes prevalent in arts work, communications, education and of course reminiscence work itself have complemented the parallel growth in person-centred and relationship-centred approaches to dementia care (Basting, 1998; Bruce, 1998; Killick & Allan, 2001).

The chapter discusses recent arts-based reminiscence initiatives which have been effective in supporting people with varying degrees of cognitive impairment, including those with little or no remaining verbal communication. The chapter shows that reminiscence work has proved to be an adaptable tool that can be used in many different situations, working with individuals at home or in care settings, and groups in the community or in day centres, care homes or supported housing.

It may initially seem paradoxical to offer memory-based activity to those whose memories are being compromised by dementing processes. How can working with a weakness create a strength? How can people develop self-confidence and a sense of identity in the present, when the memories of their own lives, their past experience, their awareness of their own past selves are apparently becoming more and more inaccessible and difficult to articulate? How can the fragmented, disjointed and increasingly misty remnants of the past be made to cohere, to create meaning and self-hood for people with dementia and those who care for them?

Reminiscence work in dementia care has consistently emphasized the importance of listening to the person, drawing them out, supporting their self-expression, connecting with them and enabling them to connect with others. The need for appropriate multi-sensory stimuli, closely matched to the person's known background and life experience, has led to the development of useful resources to trigger personal and community memories and to support workers in the dementia field (Heathcote, 2007).

Non-verbal communication tools have been developed through which people with dementia can actively participate in reminiscence programmes, sharing and showing aspects of their own remembered lives and linking successfully with others. These innovative and imaginative approaches have enabled many people with dementia to overcome some of their sense of isolation and powerlessness and to become valued members of ongoing social groups built on enjoyment and mutual acceptance. The creative approaches to communication pioneered in reminiscence and related activity groups in recent years have also enabled those who live and work with people with dementia to extend their own capacity to work creatively with, relate positively to and have fun with those in their care.

There are many different approaches to reminiscence and life story work with people with dementia, but this chapter focuses on a creative arts-based approach to reminiscence developed over many years with different groups of people (Bruce et al., 1999, Schweitzer & Bruce, 2008) and taken forward with people who have dementia in the 'Remembering Yesterday, Caring Today' project, commonly known as the RYCT project. This approach involves people with dementia and their carers as equal participants in a semi-structured series of meetings and brings the principles of person-centred dementia care (Brooker, 2004; Kitwood, 1997) to good practice in reminiscence work.

The wider context and changing attitudes to dementia

Much of the work to date in the dementia field has focused on measuring people's deficits. This is valuable in arriving at a diagnosis and enabling those affected and their families to secure services to help them cope (DH, 2009). However, the inevitable emphasis on the deteriorating capacities of the person with dementia, however tactfully expressed, can have the undesired effect of accelerating a sense of dependency, and increased stress and social isolation for all involved. The downward trajectory, which is implied or even openly predicted, when dementia is diagnosed can imbue the person with dementia and their carers with gloom, even despair and, at best, a kind of grim determination to carry on as long as is humanly possible. It can also tend to lower expectation of what life in the future has to offer and, in particular, what the person with dementia will be able to do and to enjoy.

'The curse of dementia' a phrase used in a recent British radio programme is symptomatic of how the media presents dementia and its affects. Indeed, until relatively recently, it was how the major service organizations themselves presented dementia, and it is remarkable to note how the language is gradually shifting. For example, the Alzheimer's Society in the UK in recent years has dropped the word 'Disease' from its title and moderated the 'disaster' language which used to prevail in its introductory literature for families. There is a growing emphasis on the concept of dementia as a disability which, like other disabilities, society can work with and come to terms with. People with a disability increasingly expect society to listen to them, to plan for, and with, them and to adapt to their needs. Although this is often more an aspiration than a reality, it is recognized as a standard to be worked towards.

The focus of caring organizations has, until relatively recently, been on the family carer and his or her need for moral support, hence the exponential growth in valuable support groups where carers can meet one another, share difficulties and gain strength to continue. Care of people with dementia has largely provided a kind of warehousing, to keep people safe and allow family carers some respite from their 'burden'.

A more recent emphasis has been on working with people with dementia and their carers together to support the relationship and communication between them (Cantley & Bowes, 2004; Kurokawa, 1998; Sheard, 2004). An interesting change in attitudes in the past decade has been noticeable in the annual conferences of the big organizations, such as the Alzheimer's Society and Alzheimer's International, and in their regional events and related training programmes. Carers still speak powerfully at these events but, increasingly, people with dementia themselves share their experience of having dementia. They speak of the things which make their lives difficult, but nevertheless, how it is very much worth living, and how society could adapt to give them better support and greater inclusion. At a recent Alzheimer's Society event in Belfast, the most inspiring presentation was by the Scottish Dementia Working Group who spoke up for themselves with absolute clarity, not as 'sufferers', a term they firmly rejected, but rather as a strong group with a clear vision for living life to the full despite their dementia (Scottish Dementia Working Group, 2008).

There has been recognition of the unfavourable social positioning of people with dementia and their continuing need for social inclusion and relationship (Nolan et al., 2004; Sabat, 2001). People with dementia do not exist in a closed world, even though many social avenues which used to be open to them do seem to exclude them now, or else appear too threatening or complicated for them to negotiate in their changing, less assured state. Certainly, their central relationships, whether to a life partner or other family members, do take on a greater significance at a time of increasing dependency, but there is also scope within the new situations they are facing for other and sometimes even more rewarding social relationships to develop. These new social relationships need to be relaxed and failure-free; not geared around testing of any kind (usually associated with negativity and deterioration) and not associated with clinical environments, hospitals and medical terminology.

The new social situations do not need to focus on dementia but on other aspects of life, where participants have other things in common, both in their past and current lives, as well as their present experience of living with dementia. Again, there are useful parallels with the world of disability. Activities and meetings for people with a disability used to concentrate on that disability. For example, the radical theatre groups for disabled people used to focus on sharing the experience of disability with other disabled people or conveying it to 'outsiders' in a campaigning spirit. Nowadays however, the emphasis is on normalizing disabilities as far as possible, so that disabled actors can perform in shows which are not about their disability, and wherein they can participate equally with non-disabled people, who need to make whatever (usually modest) adaptations are required for this to happen. Graeae Theatre, one of the foremost such UK companies, states its aim on its website as 'To redress the exclusion of people with physical and sensory impairments from performance and to create genuinely pioneering theatre in both its aesthetic and content.'

Reminiscence can be an equivalent 'normalizing' process in relation to dementia. Evidence shows that it is a particularly appropriate tool for linking people isolated by dementia back into the wider social fabric. A past which can be recalled and shared by all in the group, provided appropriate stimulus is offered, is a place where common ground emerges and where participants at very different levels of impairment can feel at home. The past is also a place where members of a family, and a couple in particular, were perhaps in a more equally balanced relationship, and one where tasks, responsibilities and pleasures were once shared more evenly. The recall of these times can greatly reinforce and support the husband/wife or parent/child relationship in the present when it is subject to unexpected and unwanted pressures and strains due to greater dependency levels.

Let yourself imagine a weekly reminiscence group composed of people with dementia, family carers, volunteers and a couple of skilled group leaders. Imagine an afternoon in an attractive meeting place where people have come to share memories of, for example, looking good, going out dancing and meeting someone special.

The families would have hunted down old photos, dance shoes, handbags, adverts, cinema cuttings books, love letters, favourite perfumes and anything else which might remind them and others of a time remembered quite fondly. The group leaders would have gathered objects and images to handle and talk about in small groups as people arrive, and music will be playing (ideally live, but if not on a CD or an audio tape) to evoke memories.

There will be an informal atmosphere, a personal greeting for each participant, recognizing that it has not necessarily been easy for them to get to the meeting. Some family carers will probably have come looking grey and exhausted, telling the group leaders how they were not feeling up to anything much today because of what has been going on at home.

As the session begins, people chat at small tables sharing memories, as far as possible on a one-to-one basis, handling the objects, looking at photos and singing snatches of favourite songs or dance tunes. Perhaps there will be a simple shared physical warm-up with words and actions connected to the theme, which everyone joins in. There will be an opportunity for each small group to prepare something to share with the wider group through a short improvised scene, a drawing, a collage, a shared storytelling or some other creative manifestation of the conversation which has occurred in the small groups.

Each group will listen to and look at what the others have prepared and will share further impromptu reminiscences; the people with dementia contributing perhaps a single word, a phrase or a spontaneous action, but still showing their engagement, understanding and shared experience.

There will almost certainly be some dressing up, or handling of dresses or pictures of dresses or dress patterns from their young days, and some dancing, perhaps with a bit of shared humour around how one asked partners to dance or how one politely rejected unskilled dancers who might show up. There will be tea and cakes and perhaps even a spot of alcohol. At the end of the session, there will be a recapitulation of what occurred, and some preparation for the next session, including what people can do at home in readiness, and what items they might look for to make it equally lively. There will probably be a final song and personal farewells, with quite a few hugs, appreciation for the contributions made by the people with dementia and maybe a quiet word of encouragement between carers or from the group leaders.

Most people will go home feeling that they have successfully participated in an enjoyable social event where they have had meaningful contact with others around, shared experiences and where they have been a valued member of a desirable social group. Some carers will have been genuinely surprised by how much their person has remembered and how fully he or she has participated. Anyone looking in on the group would have been challenged to spot who were the people with dementia, as the prevailing feeling had been one of fun and creativity. A further cry from the 'disaster scenario' referred to at the beginning of this section would be hard to imagine.

The 'Remembering Yesterday, Caring Today' project

I shall now describe in some detail an example of the successful use of reminiscence in dementia care with special reference to a nationally and internationally tested programme entitled 'Remembering Yesterday, Caring Today'. This project grew out of a conference entitled 'Widening Horizons in Dementia Care', organized by the European Reminiscence Network in London in 1997. It brought together thinkers and practitioners in dementia care and reminiscence specialists from Europe, United States of America, South America, Australia and Asia to share experience and to plan for the future.

Lars Rasmussen, a statistician from the health promotion wing of the European Commission in Luxembourg challenged the European Reminiscence Network to face up to the growth of dementia across Europe in the past decade and its predicted exponential growth in the next 30 years, in line with increasing life expectancy linked to rising standards of living and medical and scientific advances. He indicated that the provision of care home and nursing home places would be quite unable to keep pace, and that most caring would be delivered in the home and by family carers with some community care support. This, he suggested should be the area of focus for the European Reminiscence Network and the assembled dementia specialists. How could we create interventions which would enable carers to continue to care and which would enhance the quality of life for them and their people with dementia?

From this conference grew the RYCT project with partners in 12 countries operating pilot groups. The group leaders from participating countries trained together in London before setting up their groups, so that there would be a consistency of approach and project content. The pilot groups worked in parallel through a planned 18-week programme of activities, pursuing different topics in the life cycle each week, from earliest memories up to the present day. Up to 12 families took part in each group supported by health and social care professionals and volunteers and guided by the group leaders, many of whom had an arts and reminiscence background. All the project leaders from across Europe met to share problems and successes half-way through the cycle of sessions, and pooled results at the end.

Partners wrote up their experience of running the project (Bruce et al., 1999), showing how it had to be adapted in different countries to suit specific problems and conditions, while remaining true to the spirit of RYCT. The formal evaluation by Professor Faith Gibson, Errollyn Bruce and Dr Marianne Heinemann-Knoch (RYCT Conference Papers, 1998) endorsed the approach, indicating that there had been a high level of satisfaction from almost all participants. It was not always clear that the so-called training element had been taken on and incorporated into their lives by the family carers, so this was earmarked as a possible area for further study. However, the project had been effective in bringing the people with dementia and their carers into closer and more positive engagement with each other and others in the group, and the level of participation of people with dementia had been far greater than expected.

In some countries, the family carers were so reluctant to end the meetings that they took the initiative to continue meeting every month. One such group of carers involved in the London RYCT project created their own organization (the Reminiscence Reunion Club) and still meet a decade after the original pilot project, welcoming people from each new RYCT group to join them when their 12 weekly sessions come to an end. The most recent meeting of the London group in April 2009 attracted 50 people, people with dementia and their carers, who met to share memories around their wedding days.

At the concluding conference of the pilot RYCT project in Vienna in 1998, Lars Rasmussen again attended and issued a further challenge: 'The intervention appears to have been successful in helping the participating families and increasing their capacity to sustain positive relationships and attitudes, but how can you prove that it works, beyond anecdotal evidence and the consistently high attendance figures? What convincing evidence can you produce?'

Ever since the Vienna conference, that attempt has been ongoing, not just in Britain, but in many of the original participating European countries, including Germany, France, Sweden, Finland, Belgium, Netherlands and Austria. It has also been successfully introduced and developed in additional countries, including Spain, Italy, Greece, Romania and the Czech Republic. The RYCT project has certainly been delivered more than one hundred times. In most cases, the 18-week duration has been reduced to 12 weeks, partly for economic reasons and partly because some families have proved reluctant to commit longer to what is, after all, something of an unknown quantity. However, these 12-session projects have often given rise to the formation of Reunion groups which can run for many more months, or even years, allowing participants to remain in contact with one another and to receive continuing support from their group leaders.

In the UK, the project has attracted funding from a wide variety of sources including Allied Dunbar and Zurich Insurance Companies and the Bridge House Trust (now City Bridge Trust). In 2006–2008, the UK Medical Research Council funded a trial platform study in London, Bangor (North Wales) and Bradford involving three universities in an evaluation of the effectiveness of the RYCT intervention. The study was a controlled trial with before and after measures with both intervention groups and controls. The trial produced positive findings concerning relief of carer stress, decrease in depression and improved experience of life quality among participants when compared with controls. The Department of Health's Research Institute in the UK has now funded a more extensive study of the effectiveness (and cost effectiveness) of the RYCT intervention involving 750 people, making it the most extensive evaluation of reminiscence work attempted anywhere to date. Five university research departments are involved and will report their findings in 2011. In this ongoing study, 24 RYCT groups will run across the UK. Whatever the outcome of the study, and we all hope they will be very encouraging, the lives of many participating families coping at home with dementia will have been affected in what we hope will be a positive and significant way.

So what is distinctive about the RYCT project? It is an intervention involving people with dementia and family carers together. There have been, until quite recently, surprisingly few dementia care projects aimed at both parties in this relationship, and almost none which provide a structured programme for exploring their lived past together in the present. In the weekly sessions, the families meet others in a similar position and, instead of discussing the circumstances of their dementia, they discuss a different reminiscence topic each week following the life course from earliest memories of home and family, through school days, working life, marriage and adult family life up to the present day. Volunteers, mostly older people themselves, support the group, which may also include staff from agencies involved in providing services for people with dementia, for whom it is a valuable opportunity to learn about reminiscence.

The groups are run by skilled reminiscence workers, who have the crucial role of stimulating all the participants, structuring the sessions so that the people with dementia have maximum opportunities for successful participation and guiding the group through a pre-planned set of activities. These activities include different forms of artistic expression, such as drawing, dramatic improvisation, singing and dance. This is important as different participants respond strongly to different opportunities for expression and activity, so each session contains a balance of creative and practical work and quiet discussion time.

There is always a mixture of small-group work where one-to-one attention can be given to people who need more time to communicate, and whole group work where the insights and stories from the small groups can be more widely shared. In this way, memories and experiences which have emerged can be made available to everyone, giving special focus to different participants who would not necessarily have been able to relate their experience clearly to a large group of people themselves. Sharing the stories makes it possible for participants to find common ground for future discussions and exchanges. Perhaps it will emerge that two or three of them worked in the same place or attended the same church, cinema or dance hall, or had a shared interest in gardening, stamp collecting, sport or choral singing.

The group leaders will also facilitate some 'carers only' sessions in which they clarify the basic principles and values of RYCT. Modelling positive attitudes to people with dementia, highlighting the need to focus on successes of the people with dementia, discouraging carers from speaking negatively about their person in front of them and enabling carers to empathize through particular exercises with what it might be like to experience dementia – all these form part of these discussions. The 'carers only' sessions also provide an important place to share difficulties with other carers and gain from one another's experience. However, the group leaders' main task is to ensure that the emphasis and major focus of the work remains the reminiscence and related creative activities.

Practical guidance and directions

The approach outlined above is now formulated and well documented (Schweitzer & Bruce, 2008) but it is also constantly evolving and is extremely adaptable to suit different circumstances. This dynamic flexibility is vital as no two situations involving dementia are identical and people develop their own ways and means of coping. However, the essential elements in the project are always respected: the people with dementia are offered sensory stimulation related to the specific themes of the different sessions, a variety of activities utilizing non-verbal as well as other skills, including a range of creative activities, the chance to speak or otherwise communicate and be listened to with respect and attention and the opportunity to listen to and engage with their own and other people's memories.

It might be helpful for readers to visualize such a session in a little more detail, so that the variety of activity within a single topic is clear. Some activities in the following description might take a longer time than others, and it is likely that the group will not manage to try out all the suggestions. The group leaders running the sessions have their strengths too and will probably concentrate on the elements they feel confident they can deliver well. For this reason and to ensure a variety of approaches and styles, we have made a practice of having two group leaders with complementary skills in charge of each project. This also helps to ensure that no one is left out of conversations and activities and that one of the leaders is always watching out for anyone who may possibly become isolated unhappy or agitated.

Sample Reminiscence Session: The next generation – babies and children

Objectives

* To recall memories of looking after babies and children, and memories associated with them, such as love, playfulness, being big and strong compared to them, the smell and feel of babies, noise and movement, tickling, chasing, hide and seek, 'kissing it better' and naughtiness.
* To express opinions about something that affects everyone (we have all been cared for as babies and children, and most of us have cared for them too).
* To revisit past competence and responsibilities, and maybe remind spouses and sons and daughters who are now carers how things used to be very different.

Triggers

Old-fashioned feeding bottle, nappy, big safety pin, bibs, rattles, teddies, rose-hip oil, weighing book, national dried milk, welfare orange juice bottle, baby name book, Christening gown, matinee jacket, knitting patterns, photos of babies in old-fashioned baby clothes.

Opening

Greet people as they arrive and show them 'the new baby' (doll) in a cot or pram or cradle or in volunteer's arms (a real one would be even better!!). Everyone is invited to choose a name and sex for the baby as they come in. Leader invites each person in turn to share the name they'd give the baby and the gift they would give it as a fairy godmother (e.g. lots of love, money, a rabbit, cuddles, a locket and money).

Warm-up

Mime and copy actions relating to babies (e.g. patting and winding the baby, rocking the baby, giving medicine and smacking the toddler).

Main activities

1. Working in small groups, ask people to choose an object from the display and talk about memories associated with the item in their group, or show by their actions with the object what they associate that object with. Share stories with the whole group.
2. Remember the sayings (e.g. spare the rod and spoil the child) and the dos and don'ts of child rearing (e.g. not picking up, feeding on the hour, old wives tales, home remedies, gripe water and what to feed babies) in the whole group.

Tea break

1. Serve rusks and Ribena (and real tea as well).
2. Use the tea break to remember all the clever ways parents got their babies to eat, such as 'Down the red lane!' or 'Here comes the train into the tunnel!'
3. Return to small groups to 'bathe the baby'. Have enough bowls, dolls and towels for each family to have a go, and clothes to put on the babies after they are bathed.

Alternatively, have one bath and one doll and let people have a turn at showing their skill and methods. Encourage people to talk about memories of bathing babies, or being bathed as small children. Try out the different ways people used to fold nappies and put them on their babies, using as lifelike a doll as possible for this, to stimulate memories of texture and action/movement.

4. What has happened to the babies and children participants looked after? In small groups, each person tell about one baby or child they cared about and say what happened to them when they grew up. Maybe someone will talk about or show photos of a baby precious to them today. Share these stories with the whole group. (It is important to open up the topic to cover nieces and nephews and the children of close friends for group members who do not have their own children.)

5. Working as a whole group, remember songs sung to babies and favourite stories told to children. Invite people to sing the songs they remember to everyone, or tell the stories.

Closing

1. Leader facilitates summing-up, asking the group for their moments to remember from the session.
2. Thanks and personal goodbyes.

In some countries, where the concept of volunteering is less developed than in the UK, the groups have to run without volunteers. However, where they can be found, and appropriately trained in the principles and practice of the project beforehand, they make a tremendous contribution. The fact that they are perceived to be coming for their own enjoyment of reminiscence, and that they are clearly choosing to spend an afternoon a week with the families affected by dementia, has the effect of normalizing the meetings and making the project feel more obviously like a social than a therapeutic group. In fact, people continue to refer to 'reminiscence therapy', but the preferable terms are 'reminiscence' or 'reminiscence work'. Although the therapeutic effects of reminiscence on most participants are quite evident, it is not usually helpful to describe it as a therapy. This medical terminology rather alters the nature of the contract people enter into when they join such a group and certainly affects their expectations as to what it can achieve and their role within it.

The more attractive and non-clinical the meeting place can be for reminiscence work, the better, so that the weekly events can feel as much like a party as possible. A light room is desirable, with comfortable chairs, but not so comfortable that people will not want to get up and move around! Ideally some drapes or curtains will help improve the acoustics, which (if too echo-y) can adversely affect hearing. Facilities for making refreshments and for engaging in some 'messy' activity (such as painting, gardening and cooking) are important, and access to a piano (and a pianist!) is of course a tremendous advantage. If there is a local museum to contribute reminiscence resources from their 'handling collection' this can reduce the work load of project organizers and increase the likelihood of participants finding appealing things to handle and talk about. Proximity to public transport is very desirable and helps families feel independent in attending the project. Taxis, whether paid for or provided as a voluntary service, are preferable to minibus trips with their frequent time-consuming stops to pick people up. Many families participating in RYCT projects have developed good relationships with their taxi drivers, who themselves come to value the project as they see the beneficial effect the meetings have on their passengers.

A lot of what happens in a reminiscence group is actually an artificial recreation of what all of us do naturally when we meet our friends, especially long-standing friends. We greet them, we share memories of things we have done in the past and people we have known and we rely on them to remind us of things which connect us and which we might otherwise have forgotten. Our meetings are successful when we have a meaningful exchange on a fairly equal basis, with some laughter, some understanding and mutual sympathy concerning sad memories, which will inevitably come up, and possibly even some disagreements with one another, which we can live with pretty comfortably. After such meetings we feel more in touch, not just with our old friends but also with ourselves. We will have re-established the link between our present selves and our younger selves, between our life in the present and the many different stages of the long life we have led. As some of the remembered energy and competence of our younger selves is reawakened through our sharing of memories it can help us to feel more alive and more confident in the present, more a 'whole person' and better equipped to face the future.

For older people in general, who may have lost track of very long-standing close friends and relations, and for older people with dementia in particular, such meetings in the course of normal life are rarities. They need to be artificially engineered by creating groups specifically for that purpose and ensuring that the structures are in place for locating and sharing memories and generating new relationships. This is exactly why RYCT can work for people with dementia and their carers where the sessions, each of which has a specific topic around which most people have experience, can enable people to find others with common interests and experience. People exchange memories with other group members, often of a similar age and background, and in so doing, they build new present-day friendships through their memories, and they also relocate their younger and sometimes more confident selves as they bring their pasts into the present. Don, a family carer in a recent RYCT group commented about his wife: What I did find was that the more we got into this course, she used to get a bit stroppy with me. After coming here, if I was cooking the evening meal, she'd come out and say, 'You know you're not doing that properly. You're not doing it the way I'd do it.' So it did improve her self-confidence and then she wouldn't take kindly to being told what to do all the time.

We have discovered that even people who cannot speak themselves, and are unable to tell their own stories, nevertheless enjoy joining in vicariously as they listen to their family carer telling stories about them from earlier times. In fact the carer has an important role here, to enable the rest of the group to visualize and get to know their person as they were before they developed dementia. One carer who spoke about her own and her partner's life reported that the process was particularly important for her because it put the present rather testing situation in the longer context of a shared lifetime. She was able to reflect back on the many changes in fortune and

ways of overcoming difficulties with which she and her partner had successfully coped in the past and to gain strength to
manage the present as a resourceful and experienced adult.

Bob, another carer commented on how important it was for
him to hold onto the past in the marriage to sustain him in
the present: 'I found that my recollections would be coloured
by the day-to-day life to such an extent that I would bury the
past. So I sat down and I wrote for myself, and ultimately
for the children, a brief account of how Helga and I met and
tried to paint a picture of her as she was then. And I did that,
but I still have this feeling that the longer you live with this
present state, the thicker the glass gets between you and what
was once a clear picture. I find I cannot always access the past
myself. For me it's hazy. This (RYCT) activity sometimes
sparks memory. When it's just come into your mind, it's fresh
for a little while, something that might not otherwise have
come. In that sense, this has been very useful.'

Conclusion and the way forward

In the UK the use of reminiscence is increasingly becoming
embedded in dementia care and dementia organizations. Tom
Kitwood was very clear about the value of knowing the person's life story (Kitwood, 1997) in understanding each person's
individuality and giving appropriate care. Reminiscence, which
involves exploring the person's life experience and attitudes has fit-
ted comfortably alongside other positive dementia care initiatives
and has been an element in many research approaches, including cognitive stimulation (Spector et al., 2006), social engagement (Brooker, 2007), social and emotional support (Jones and
Miesen, 2004) life history work (Bruce & Schweitzer, 2008;
Stokes, 2008) and Life Review (Haight & Webster, 1995).

The active listening to the person and the feeding back
of what they have said are important elements not only in
reminiscence work but also in any kind of communication.
Ideas for conversation borrowed from the project outline have
proved useful to people in very different situations, such as in
understanding unaccountable behaviour (Schweitzer & Bruce,
2008) and in making activities in daily living more pleasurable

(Gibson, 2004). When bathing, dressing or feeding an individual, for example, it has been found helpful to exchange stories about washing and dressing in the past and it has enabled a more active involvement of the person in, for example, choosing what to wear or what to eat.

The RYCT project has proved to be very adaptable and ideas from it have been followed in non-community settings where the person with dementia is already in residential or nursing care. It has considerable potential for involving friends and relatives of people admitted to care homes in being able to continue to share the care of their relative and to find meaningful roles within their inevitably altered circumstances. People who have cared for someone at home often feel a profound sense of regret and even failure when their person goes into residential care (Woods et al., 2007, 2008). Reminiscence groups are an invaluable way of bringing these ex-carers into the life of the home. They can help their person to tell their stories and thereby help the staff to know them in a more personal way and care for as individuals. Relatives can also meet other residents and family members, thus helping the facility to become an open caring community. A future research project is currently in the planning stages to explore further the use of RYCT in care homes with support from relatives.

For those of us who have been involved in the development of the project over a number of years, it has been immensely encouraging to see how widely it has been accepted as an accessible and enjoyable, low-risk intervention. It is hoped that the current rigorous research will confirm the indicative findings of the earlier small pilot studies and that acceptable evidence of effectiveness will be established.

The main purpose of RYCT remains to give families coping with dementia an opportunity to restore, renew, enrich or create a closer bond between their own members and to make new and lasting links with other families through sharing significant memories and engaging in enjoyable memory-related creative reminiscence activities together. It is designed to support crucial relationships and to help participating families to re-access the great reserves of goodwill that have sustained their relationships over the years. Even for those who look back with less equanimity and whose relationships are more problematic, this project does offer a chance to support their person in making contact with others and remembering better times together.

References

Basting, A. (1998). *The Stages of Age*. Michigan: University of Michigan Press.

Brooker, D. (2004). What is person-centred care? *Reviews in Clinical Gerontology*, 13(3), 215–222.

Brooker, D. (2007). *Person-Centred Dementia Care: Making Services Better*. London: Jessica Kingsley.

Bruce, E. (1998). Reminiscence and Family Carers. In P. Schweitzer (ed.), *Reminiscence in Dementia Care*. London: Age Exchange.

Bruce, E., Hodgson, S. & Schweitzer, P. (1999). *Reminiscing with People with Dementia: A Handbook for Carers*. London: Age Exchange (for the European Reminiscence Network).

Bruce, E. & Schweitzer, P. (2008). Working with Life History. In M. Downs & B. Bowers (eds), *Excellence in Dementia Care*. Maidenhead: McGraw Hill.

Cantley, C. & Bowes, A. (2004). Dementia and Social Inclusion: The Way Forward. In A. Innes, C. Archibald & C. Murphy (eds), *Dementia and Social Inclusion*. London: Jessica Kingsley.

Conference Papers of European Reminiscence Network, *Remembering Yesterday, Caring Today: Reminiscence, People with Dementia and their Family Carers*, Vienna, November 1998.

DH (2009). *Living Well with Dementia: A National Dementia Strategy*. (dh.gov.uk/en/Publicationsandstatistics/Publications/.../DH_094058 accessed 21 July 2009).

Gibson, F. (2004). *The Past in the Present: Using Reminiscence in Health and Social Care*. Baltimore: Health Professions Press.

Haight, B. & Webster, J. (1995). *The Art and Science of Reminiscing*. Washington: Taylor & Francis.

Heathcote, J. (2007). *Memories Are Made of This: Reminiscence Activities for Person-Centred Care*. London: Alzheimer's Society. http://www.graeae.org/.

Jones, G. & Miesen, B. (2004). *Caregiving in Dementia: Research and Applications, Volume 3*. London: Brunner/Routledge.

Killick, J. & Allan, K. (2001). *Communication and the Care of People with Dementia*. Buckingham: Open University Press.

Kitwood, T. (1997). *Dementia Reconsidered: The Person Comes First.* Buckingham: Open University Press.

Kurakawa, Y. (1998). Couple Reminiscence with Japanese Dementia Patients. In P. Schweitzer (ed.). *Reminiscence in Dementia Care.* London: Age Exchange.

Nolan, M., Davies, S. J., Brown, J., Keady, J. & Nolan, J. (2004). Beyond 'person-centred care': a new vision for gerontological nursing. *International Journal of Older People Nursing* in association with *Journal of Clinical Nursing,*13 (3a), 45–53.

Sabat, S. (2001). *Life through a Tangled Veil: The Experience of Alzheimer's Disease.* Oxford: Blackwell.

Schweitzer, P. & Bruce, E. (2008). *Remembering Yesterday, Caring Today: Reminiscence in Dementia Care.* London: Jessica Kingsley.

Scottish Dementia Working Group (2008). *What disempowers us – and what can be done* website Alzheimer Scotland, www.sdwg.org.uk.

Sheard, D. (2004). Bringing relationships into the heart of dementia care. *Journal of Dementia Care,* 12(4), 22–24.

Spector, A. Thorgrimsen, L. Woods, B. and Orrell, M. (2006). *Making a Difference: an Evidence-Based Group Programme to Offer Cognitive Stimulation Therapy (CST) to People with Dementia.* Hawker Publications: UK.

Stokes, G. (2008). *And Still the Music Plays: Stories of People with Dementia.* London: Hawker Publications.

Woods, B., Keady, J. & Seddon, D. (2007). *Involving Families in Care Homes: A Relationship-Centred Approach to Dementia Care.* London: Jessica Kingsley Publishers.

Woods, B., Keady, J. & Seddon, D. (2008). *Partners in Care (30 Minute Video).* London: Jessica Kingsley Publishers.

10 Getting in the picture: using photography, video and visual material to enhance communication

John Killick and Kate Allan

Introduction

> After many years of wandering in the wilderness I was diagnosed with dementia. Before and after that I had spent my time at home deeply distressed and unable to function. I had hit rock bottom. Marilyn, a skilled photographer, encouraged me to start taking photos again. I had forgotten how to use my camera and needed retraining. I had previously only taken snaps of the children growing up but now I looked at things in a new light and tried to produce photos which reflected not the stark image of the subject but rather a mood. I feel it is important that the photos show what can be achieved when a person is given person-centred help.

These are the words of James McKillop (McKillop, 2003), a man from Glasgow with a diagnosis of early onset dementia, who found a sense of purpose and an outlet for his creative impulses in taking photographs. He is not alone in having found a new way forward through the use of photography and video.

We believe that the sensitive use of visual media can help people with dementia in a variety of ways: to stay creative or to discover their creativity for the first time, to reinforce and develop personal identity, to boost confidence and self-esteem through having opportunities to take control and make choices, to experience positive emotion and enhance well-being and to provide whole new arenas for communication.

We have so much to learn from people with dementia about what it means to live with this condition. For us all the opportunity to create images and films means we can show others what is important to us and how the world looks from our point of view. For the person with dementia who is making a journey through a multitude of transitions and challenges, created both by the condition and the responses of those around them, the opportunity to use photography and video to share their experience can be empowering and enlightening and has the potential to change things for the better in important ways.

We begin this chapter by exploring why working with images and film has so much positive potential for people with dementia. We then look at a number of examples which are showing us the way, beginning with the process of creating photographs. We then consider the activity of making films. Finally we look at the possibilities of working with existing images and films to enhance the lives of people with the condition. We do not consider the subject of reminiscence in this chapter, although much of what we talk about is potentially applicable to this sphere of activity.

The advantages of visual media for people with dementia

People with dementia often experience changes in their usual ways of communicating, and in our highly verbal culture they may find themselves seriously disadvantaged in expressing themselves and engaging with others. Visual imagery is largely independent of words, and therefore offers particularly powerful ways of communicating for persons who find that using language has become difficult.

We also know that dementia is often associated with difficulties in the area of logical, linear thinking. Again pictorial media provide an alternative and rich way of presenting or conveying information, acting as a 'meeting point' for shared experience and communication.

For many people, with or without dementia, pictures, photographs and films have an immediacy in sensory, intuitive and emotional terms which is again not dependent on cognitive pathways. As a consequence they have a special power to stimulate feelings and memories, and arouse associations. Visual images often have an ambiguous quality which invites interpretation or speculation, and appeals to the imagination. Throughout our lives we are all engaged in a search for meaning, patterns and ways of explaining what happens to us. Pictures and other visual media can help us to do this. Images can help us to piece together a story and give shape to the flux. They can also surprise, shock, charm and enthral with instances of the new, jolting us out of conventional ways of seeing and imagining.

Another advantage of visual material is its sheer availability and accessibility. We are surrounded by pictures of all sorts. Newspapers, magazines, junk mail and the Internet are full of them, in addition to more personal items such as an individual's own possessions. Further, the means for creating new pictures is becoming ever more accessible and easy to use: low-cost disposable cameras, together with the profusion of digital tools, means that it has never been easier or cheaper to create images, and to manipulate and personalize them. Although the older individuals in the current population of people with dementia may be less familiar with such means, people who have developed their condition more recently are likely to have the experience of using digital technology through either work or leisure.

A word of caution: working with visual media will not suit everyone. As we learn more about the nature of their condition, we are coming to understand that some people with dementia experience profound changes in their way of perceiving and interpreting visual stimuli. Indeed some have gone as far as to say that dementia should be understood as a 'visuo-perceptual' disability, as well as an intellectual one (Miesen & Jones, 2006). For such individuals it may be confusing or distressing to try to enter into a more visually orientated world.

Making photographs and other images

The opening quotation from James McKillop illustrates how meaningful photography became for him. Cameras, simple and sophisticated, offer us an opportunity to capture a moment in time and to keep it, something which has a powerful appeal to us all. For the individual with dementia, who is living with memory loss and confusion, such an opportunity may take on an even deeper and more poignant significance.

In her resource *(which includes books and CD Rom)*, *Focusing on the Person*, about the potential of photography for people with dementia, Occupational Therapist Claire Craig encourages us to appreciate the many ways in which photography can play a positive role in the person's life. There is a great deal of practical advice, including discussion of the various options in terms of the types of cameras which can be used, their advantages and limitations and the particular challenges that a person with dementia might encounter. Sometimes the person will have their own camera and be comfortable using it. Also, the option of using disposable film cameras which are extremely simple to operate is very accessible. Digital photography, as the now dominant method, varies widely in terms of sophistication. Most mobile phones have integrated cameras meaning that basic photographs can be taken at a moment's notice. The simplest of dedicated digital cameras are very cheap and can be used with the most basic type of computer which will normally come loaded with software to do basic image processing, such as viewing and cropping. Printing can be done either with one's own printer or is available very cheaply in photography shops. The range of options for working with digital images is increased hugely with the help of software which allows for altering aspects of the photograph, such as brightness and contrast and colour balance. Often such software is preloaded on computers or can be obtained for no cost. More sophisticated software allows for a further and truly dizzying array of options.

Claire also discusses the possibilities in terms of where to go and what to photograph, and provides suggestions for what to do with the resulting images (considered in more detail later in the chapter). As always, her emphasis is on understanding the ways in which a particular activity, such as photography, can be used to meet the individual person's needs. For example, it may be about having the opportunity to make choices, to tell a story or to have enjoyment and fun. Putting the person's needs at the forefront and adapting the way we approach an activity helps to ensure that we are providing truly person-centred care, rather than just shoehorning individuals into a more standardized format.

The emphasis on meeting needs also reminds us that although we tend to look at the resulting image as the most important aspect of photography, as with all creative work involving people with dementia, it is vital to focus on the value of the *process*. In photography there is the experience of inter-acting with others, handling a camera, going to locations to take pictures, looking at what is to be photographed, having the opportunity to make decisions and judgements, the satisfaction of capturing something, the anticipation of seeing the resulting images and the impact of re-encountering the original subject in its captured form, together with the discussion of the experience with the expression of feelings and memories.

Claire describes the experience of working with one man as follows:

> The photographs certainly weren't beautiful in an aesthetic sense. Picture after picture striking only in their ordinariness. Onlookers might easily have passed over them, dismissing their significance, but when you had been there, sharing every step of the way with Harry, his complete concentration, repeating over and over again the simple instructions necessary to operate the camera, well then the photographs took on a different significance, a whole new meaning. Every detail contained in those images had been considered and deliberate. I had observed every moment with complete fascination and through this process we had developed a shared understanding about what was important to the both of us. The selection of coloured prints therefore represented much more than an end-result, a product to be admired by others, they were the embodiment of the journey we had travelled over time and the relationship that we had forged because of it. (Craig, 2005, p. 3)

A very successful and instructive photography initiative involving people with dementia was the 'Captured Memories' project which took place in Stirling in 2004 led by Rosas Mitchell. It was an experimental venture which explored the experience of having people with dementia take a much more active role than usual in recording a day trip photographically.

The work itself, and a book and an article (Mitchell, 2005a, 2005b) which followed, have much to teach us about the creative and communicative possibilities as well as good practice in this area. The project was based in a drop-in centre at the centre of the town, but the work was mainly done during excursions further afield. Rosas, the arts-worker, planned the initiative meticulously.

First came the preparatory stage, which itself was a highly interactive process, involving persons with dementia, relatives, friends, volunteers and a paid member of the staff. Discussions about the idea of using an excursion to a local place of historical interest as an opportunity to do a photography project took place and led to nine persons with dementia opting to take part, three of whom were wheelchair users. The factors which most influenced these individuals were confidence in their own abilities, previous experience with a camera and good relationship with a volunteer.

The next stage was in two parts. First, a trial run gave everyone confidence for the main event by providing opportunities for participants and volunteers to practice taking pictures, and to find out what the challenges and possibilities were. For the main event, lessons from the trial were put into action and each person was allocated a volunteer who supported them in whatever ways they required. According to their needs and preferences some people used disposable film cameras, some used digital ones.

Stage three involved individual interviews with all who had taken part. The in-depth discussions explored how it had felt for participants to have the opportunity to take pictures, why they had chosen specific subjects and what they thought of the outcome. This proved rich ground for reflection and reminiscence. As Rosas says

> The photos evoked a very positive reaction which brought tremendous energy into the room. People became animated, full of stories, in touch with themselves and communicating in a very lively way. Spontaneous memories came tumbling thick and fast, recalling partners, children, friends, childhood adventures and holidays, parents and operations. One woman sang through many of her playground verses. Others talked about photos bringing back sad as well as happy memories. (Mitchell, 2005b, p. 14)

Individuals responded in their own characteristic ways. Rosas comments that one man

> needed three different one-hour sessions to really sort his photo-graphs the way he wanted. He was concerned with sequence, per-sistent in problem-solving, logical in thought and concentrated until he succeeded. (Mitchell, 2005a, p. 17)

The last phase was, perhaps surprisingly, the most exten-sive. The photographs became a resource, referred back to and reused constantly in a variety of contexts. They became the focus for discussion and reminiscence, were used in craft ses-sions to make pictures and collages and were modified using stencils, cutting out, die-stamping and fabric printing. The wall displays were a wonder to behold. In addition, each pho-tographer created their own scrapbook/journal.

The staff and volunteers agreed that increase in self-esteem was the most significant gain for participants. Rosas summed the project up in the words:

> (It) shifted the balance of power, took us all out of our 'comfort zones' and helped people become more dynamic and alive. *(Mitchell, 2005b, p. 14)*

Amongst the participants' comments were the following:

> I'm tickled that I took that photo. I was very thankful that you set me up in business. I think I should become a photographer. *(Mitchell, 2005a, pp. 17–19)*

This was a model creative photography project: thoroughly planned, resourceful and life-enhancing for all concerned.

As well as providing an opportunity for creative expres-sion, photography can play an essential and very practical part in the lives of people with dementia. It can preserve information and support memory. Agnes Houston has early onset of Alzheimer's and lives in the West of Scotland. Here she describes the lifeline that photography has become for her:

> I never used the camera, then when I heard about James's (McKillop) photography I thought...what a tool! I have my camera in my bag, I

carry it everywhere, and if I want to recall somewhere I take a photograph of it. Before Christmas I had wee photographs of people I wanted to remember. So though I thought my camera was going to be used artistically like James's, it has become almost like my writing tool, a substitute for a part of the brain that's not working. (Houston in Allan & Killick, 2009)

As we noted at the start of the chapter, one role for photography is to enable an individual to present their view of the world, one that is perhaps especially important for those who are marginalized and excluded. This particular use of photography is not well-developed in relation to people with dementia, but an unusual documentary photography project involving people with dementia did touch on this role (Fleming & Uchide, 2004). The project was a collaboration between two nursing homes, one in Australia and one in Japan. It was an attempt to capture in visual terms something of the values underpinning the care in each facility. Over a few days, people with dementia, staff and relatives were encouraged to take pictures of what was important to them about each care home. Over three days no fewer than 1600 pictures were taken. All groups then participated in a process that eventually resulted in 15 pictures of each facility being included in a book called *Images of Care: Emerging Common Values*. The photographs from Japan were accompanied by a caption which provided some explanation of the picture. This was not done for the Australian images. Although we do not know which of the final images were taken by persons with dementia, the project serves as an example of what is possible in terms of conveying messages about people's lives and their feelings about them.

And as a development of her interest in photography with older people, Claire Craig is currently undertaking research in this area, working with the residents of a care home who, with her support, 'have been capturing aspects of their day to day lives on film, sharing their past and present and their hopes and wishes for the future' (Craig, 2010).

We finish this section by sharing John's experience of one lady who seemed to have an especially highly developed visual imagination, and who reminds us to take more care to notice, appreciate and celebrate the beauty in what surrounds us. She

lived in a dementia unit in a nursing home and he made a
poem from her words:

> The scenery of this room, does it ever get changed? Some of the com-
> positions are so good it would be tragic to part with them. Someone
> should photograph them before they get changed, or they could be
> lost for ever. But at the same time you need variety, don't you, or
> you've nothing to compare? People think you need something beau-
> tiful to make a picture, but what you need is skill. This room should
> be filmed before it is too late. (Killick, 2008, p. 37)

Making videos

Between 1999 and 2003, Sitar Rose, an independent documentary film-maker, was commissioned by Dementia Services
Development Centre (DSDC) at the University of Stirling to
make a series of short films in collaboration with individuals
with dementia in various care settings in and around Edinburgh.
There was no 'crew' involved so Sitar assumed the roles of inter-
viewer, camera operator and sound-recordist simultaneously.
This was demanding but ensured a degree of intimacy essential
to the process. Each person was consulted about the approach
adopted, the subjects covered, the setting(s) in which the filming
took place and any music used. Some of the portraits became life
stories based on family photographs, supplemented by footage
(with or without the person present) of significant places; others
were portrayals of life in the present, for example featuring an
encounter with a horse, thoughts and feelings about objects or a
conducted tour of *the person's home*.

Editing was carried out by Sitar herself, but again participants were involved in decisions about what to use and what to
discard, and sometimes the process of reviewing material was
filmed as well. Sitar kept a journal of each interaction, and here
is an extract from an entry:

> In amongst a lot of distraction of tea, staff and other residents show-
> ing interest in what we were doing, Irene was able to let me know
> which shots were good. She had asked me at the beginning how I
> would go about deciding what to film. I had talked about composition
> and later she started to talk about a particular shot. She said about
> one close-up of the gold chain round her neck, that it wasn't complete,

and I explained to her that I hadn't included her head because she had her rollers in and I thought she wouldn't like that.... She also admired my ring and talked quite specifically about how it was constructed, enough for me to ask her if she had ever made jewellery. She said she had. When I edit I will have to hold shots still and for a long time so that there is time for Irene to look at them and really see what is happening. The editing must be straightforward and include establishing shots to give her sufficient time to understand the images. (Rose, 2006, p. 24)

When each film was completed it was given to the person for them to do whatever they wished with it. Most of the participants were proud of their films and enjoyed seeing them, sometimes many times over. They appeared to come up fresh each time, and to have the effect of confirming for them a sense of identity. Some gave permission for the videos to be shared more widely, and three of these were published (Video Portraits, DSDC). Close relatives of the people were also involved in such a decision. In some instances relatives were not willing for them to be shared with others.

Sitar Rose makes the following general comment on the project:

The video work is a process of rediscovering the person frequently hidden by the dementia and is in no way an exposé of what effect dementia has had on the person. These are not films 'about dementia'. For the person themselves, their relatives, friends or carers, it can be a surprise to know that it might be possible for this person to emerge at a time when dementia may be inhibiting their ability to communicate quite severely. (Rose, 2006, p. 23)

And drawing attention to the unique nature of each film she says

Every video has produced a special characteristic and contains memorable moments of joy, pain, humour and reflection. One of my favourite examples is where Irene, contemplating a carved gourd in her hand, said 'That's where it is now.... but where is it in reality?' (Rose, 2006, p. 24)

The Video Portraits are sophisticated pieces of work, but there is no reason why more simple films could not be created by those in a supporting role working collaboratively with a person with dementia. Many people now own video cameras (or digital cameras with video functions), and attempting one-to-one work with individuals is well within the bounds of possibility. Similarly making a short film with a group does not necessarily require a professional. Choosing an aspect of life common to all the members or improvising a sketch gives real opportunities for creativity, bonding and enjoyment.

In 2000, a video-artist working in a care home in Stirling with staff and residents made a very successful little film entitled 'Who Am I?' The title and concept came from the participants and they adopted a very straightforward format. The ten-minute film presented a series of 'talking heads' of staff and service users, who answered a series of questions in quick succession, covering date and place of birth, and likes and dislikes in terms of food, reading and music. The whole process formed a powerful indictment of labels and barriers, conveying the message that everyone taking part was an individual with distinct personality and tastes and communication style. The enterprise had been a model in social inclusiveness and the finished film existed to carry the message far beyond the confines of the service.

Ethical considerations

Any involvement with people who are in any way more vulnerable or less powerful than ourselves demands that we operate according to high ethical standards, and activities involving photography and video call for some particular considerations. As always we must be concerned with establishing that the people involved are willing, especially if they themselves are being photographed or filmed. We all have feelings about how we wish to be portrayed and encountering what seems to us to be a bad photo can be very painful. We must also be alert to issues of confidentiality in this regard. Another type of ethical consideration revolves around issues of ownership of any images of footage, and the use of these after the activity. Addressing such concerns will involve careful communication and consultation, conducted on an ongoing basis with the individuals involved, and sometimes with their relatives.

Further consideration of ethical issues involved in the use of video (many of the lessons will also apply to photography) can be found in Cook (2002) and Knight (2005) and more generally in relation to the issue of consent to participate in activities in Allan (2001).

Using photographs and video

Most people respond to the stimulus of a familiar photograph or an unfamiliar image which is interesting, funny or beautiful, and people with dementia are no different. An album of family snaps can stir memories and emotions powerfully, and a well-chosen visual image can often prompt a response from someone who otherwise appears withdrawn. Many older people with dementia are physically limited and no longer able to visit places of which they are fond. Photographs can bring those scenes before them again.

Between 1998 and 2000, Kate ran a project exploring ways to communicate with persons with dementia in care settings, in particular consulting people about their views of services. Kate's role was to support frontline staff in their workplaces attempting small-scale innovations with individuals in their care. A variety of approaches were tried out and one of the most successful involved the use of visual materials (Allan, 2001).

Many different sorts of pictures were used, and these were collected from various sources, including in some instances the participant's own possessions. Attempts were made to find photographs which were likely to be of particular interest to the person concerned. Pictures were often used in quite general ways, for example by establishing a link with the person, who was encouraged to respond in whatever way seemed natural. For some the pictures appeared to act as a stimulus for talking about someone or something else, or encouraging relaxation and reducing any apprehension. This may well have been true of the staff too.

Sometimes looking at a picture prompted the telling of a story. As well as learning about what was important or memorable to the person, such an opportunity could give staff clues about the conversational style of the individual, for example how they used words and expressions. Photographs of objects, such as household furniture or utensils, were often used, and in one instance a photograph of dominoes resulted in the participant commenting on her enjoyment of that game; her key worker was then able to incorporate that activity in her daily routine.

One way of using photographs of people not known to the individual, for example images from magazines or newspapers, was intended to encourage participants to talk about services in an indirect way. So instead of asking a person their opinion directly, a photograph would be presented and the participant <u>was</u> invited to speculate on what the person in the picture might think or feel. Pictures were sometimes used with groups accompanied by brief vignettes composed by staff which pointed people towards certain themes or predicaments which could then be explored in discussion. Both individual and group approaches led to some very interesting reflections which seemed very unlikely to have arisen in any other way.

An organization called 'Pictures to Share' has made a valuable contribution to the use of visual media to give pleasure and stimulation, and to develop and reinforce relationships with people with dementia. This company is producing a series of large, high-quality, hardback books which are designed for long-lasting use. Each book takes a theme, such as women's work, sport, childhood, the countryside, providing a series of photographs in colour or black-and-white as triggers for interaction. The pictures are chosen for variety and excellence and are reproduced on the right-hand pages at a size of 28 by 25 cms. The opposite page is left largely blank apart from an apposite short quotation in large print. The books can be enjoyed by individuals with dementia on their own or in the company of others. The following quotation from Professor Christine E. King (from a letter to the publishers) describes this:

I bought your books for Bill, my Dad who lives with me, is 91 and has dementia. He used to love reading but has lost all interest and the ability to make sense even of illustrations. I had tried children's books but they were clearly not of interest. Your books absolutely fascinate him. He reads them every day and shows everyone who visits. The carers read through them with him daily and his depression is lifting. He says he feels 'normal' again now he can read. Thank you so much!

Jim Ellis, whose wife has dementia, has written an article about the use of photographs. Over a considerable period he collected photographs (including the 'Pictures to Share' books) to use with his wife and with other residents of a care home. He affirms that

> pictures can be highly stimulating for people with dementia but a large selection of images needs to be offered to accommodate so many unique lives. And an essential feature is the sharing of an experience that is enriching for both parties within a binding companionship. (Ellis, 2007, p. 34)

A project based on the creative use of photographs is 'Timeslips' developed in the United States by Anne Basting (2009). This is a group activity which focuses on storytelling and the use of the imagination, but is not reliant on cognitive processes of recall. All participants in a group are given copies of the same photograph and are asked a series of open-ended questions, for example 'Who is this person?' and 'What is happening?'. No contribution is rejected, and all are treated as of equal worth. During the session it is typical for a rich collection to be amassed, which are written down by one of the facilitators. Through a process of negotiation a final version of the written piece is developed, and then read back to the group, and owned by the members. The stories often reflect the hopes and fears and humour of the participants. John has practised a method of making poems with a group which follows a similar format and often results in forms of words which are highly valued by the members. As in 'Timeslips', the images are specially chosen for their potential for eliciting a variety of responses.

John also has experience of using a combination of videos and photographs in planned groups sessions. The following account comes from a report (Killick, 2006) of one such project in a day centre, which typically involved six participants in one of two groups. The activity took place in a room separate from the rest of the centre. The room was darkened for the video extracts. There were four sessions with each group, and each session lasted for approximately 50 minutes. During the sessions three video extracts were shown and four photographs discussed. The video extracts or photographs were not specifically chosen for their potential to stir memories.

> There was a similar pattern of development of involvement in both groups. By the fourth session it was increasingly difficult for me to keep to the plan I had for the session because the contributions from the participants became more fulsome, and there were far more interchanges. Indeed, by the second session with each group everyone was playing a full part. One lady in Group Two had been coming to the centre for three years and had never settled in a group before.

> The two groups developed different personalities. Group One decided early on to play things for humour. Lunch-time, which immediately followed what I had called 'Going to the Pictures', was often the occasion for comments on what had occurred. 'That's what he's here for – to make us laugh', and 'We've been working hard laughing this morning' were two such. One lady, speaking of me, said loudly 'He's not quite as stupid as he looks!'

> Group Two took a more serious approach. I showed a collage made by Ray Maloney entitled 'Blues in the Night'. One man commented 'I know exactly how he feels. I fell off a bridge and injured my head. It affected my memory badly, but it is gradually returning. It is helped by times like this.'

> I learned that it doesn't much matter what visual material you choose to present so long as it is bold and clear. A couple of the video extracts I used proved too complex for people to unravel. And the photographs mustn't be too ambiguous. The fact that none of the subjects was familiar did not seem to matter. Anyone who wished to reminisce could do so: one lady even related a photograph of an elephant in India to her childhood park in Edinburgh! And you must be prepared for the most unlikely associations to be triggered. As another lady said 'Something in that film just started me off.' (Killick, 2006, p. 33)

Here there was a sense of occasion which transformed an ordinary day into something special. There was enjoyment which released tensions and encouraged participation, bringing otherwise isolated individuals into relationship. There was creativity, in this case manifesting itself in rich, imaginative interpretation and appreciation of the material presented. There was encountering the world beyond the narrow confines of individuals with the diagnosis, and humour in which the uniqueness of individuals shone. Above all, there was the exercise of communication skills in the to-and-fro of human interaction.

Further creative processes

In addition to the range of ways in which photographs and pictures can be used as they are, it is worth mentioning the fact that of course pictorial material can be used as a starting point for further creative processes. In *Focusing on the Person*, Claire Craig (2005) provides a large number of suggestions for using photographs in the course of creating items, such as bookmarks, handmade books and calendars and also as a link into other types of creative activity such as writing and music. She also discusses ways in which photographs can play a part in the person's day-to-day care, such as illustrating preferences. The CD Rom which forms part of the resource both inspires and guides users through the practical steps.

One way of recycling pictures is to create new pictures made from them – an art form usually called collage. The process of collecting and studying existing images in order to select from them to make something new has been highly meaningful to Ray Maloney, a man with dementia who lived in Michigan. As he described it, the process of taking fragments to create a new image seemed to mirror in some way the changes he experienced as part of his condition. On a website featuring his work the following statement appears:

> Approximately three years following his diagnosis, Ray began designing collages. He usually began by painting the background in acrylics. He spent hours looking through magazines searching for images that could be used. From the thousands and thousands of pieces he cut, Ray then glued little pieces to form a collage reflecting his thoughts about living with cognitive impairment. The little pieces of paper were symbolic of the changes that were occurring in Ray's brain. (Optimal Dementia Care, 2010)

Ray had been an artist prior to developing dementia, so his collages are unusually sophisticated, but the creative arrangement of pictorial material by individuals or groups can prove a rewarding and beneficial activity more generally.

Conclusion

The opportunities for involving people with dementia in activities using photography and video are there for the taking. These art forms are so available and so malleable that they can fit naturally into ordinary routines. We believe that they should be considered an integral part of any approach for enriching the lives of those with the condition, and developing our understanding of what it means to live with it.

We end with another quote:

> When I sit here sorting through photographs, deciding what should go where, I feel that my world makes sense and I am no longer frightened.' These words were spoken (during the act of sorting through a box of photographs) by a person who had memory difficulties and severe perceptual problems. Whilst engaging in a similar activity, another person with dementia said: 'See, I've put everything in its proper slot. (Craig, 2005, p. 14)

References

Allan, K. (2001). *Communication and Consultation: Exploring Ways for Staff to Involve People with Dementia in Developing Services*. Bristol: Policy Press, (available to download from http://www.jrf.org.uk/publications/exploring-ways-staff-consult-people-with-dementia-about-services) (accessed on 16 January 2011).

Allan, K. & Killick, J. (2009). 'Making things more real': changing the way we see dementia. *Journal of Dementia Care*, 17(6), 20–21.

Basting, A. (1998). Timeslips www.timeslips.org

Basting, A.D. (2009). *Forget Memory: Creating Better Lives for people with Dementia*. Baltimore: The Johns Hopkins University.

Cook, A. (2002). Using Video Observation to Include the Experiences of People with Dementia in Research. In H. Wilkinson (ed.),*The Perspectives of People with Dementia: Research Methods and Motivations*. London: Jessica Kingsley.

Craig, C. (2005). *Focusing on the Person: Exploring the Potential of Photography for People with Dementia*. Stirling: Dementia Services Development Centre.

Craig, C. (2010) http://research.shu.ac.uk/lab4living/phd-claire-craig (accessed on 16 January 2011).

Ellis, J. (2007). Sharing pictures in a nursing home. *Signpost*, 12(2), 33–35.

Fleming, R. & Uchide, Y. (2004). *Images of Care in Australia and Japan: Emerging Common Values*. Stirling: Dementia Services Development Centre.

Killick, J. (2006). Going to the pictures: using visual media in a day centre. *Signpost*, 11(1), 32–33.

Killick, J. (2008). *Dementia Diary*. London: Hawker.

Knight, R. (2005). Interviewing people with dementia using video. *Journal of Dementia Care*, 13(3), 31–35.

McKillop, J. (2003). *Opening Shutters – Opening Minds*. Stirling: Dementia Services Development Centre.

Miesen, B. M. L & Jones, G. M. M. (2006). *Caregiving in Dementia: Research and Applications*. London: Routledge.

Mitchell, R. (2005a). *Captured Memories*. Stirling: Dementia Services Development Centre.

Mitchell, R. (2005b). I'm tickled I took that photo. *Journal of Dementia Care*, 13(2), 14.

Optimal Dementia Care http://optimaldementiacare.com/gallery.html (accessed 6 April 2010).

Pictures to Share www.picturestoshare.co.uk (accessed on 16 January 2011).

Rose, S. (2006). Video portraits: creating lasting records. *Journal of Dementia Care*, 14(5), 23–24.

11 Creative processes to bring out expressions of spirituality: working with people who have dementia

Elizabeth MacKinlay

Introduction

What's it like to be diagnosed with dementia? For more than a decade, as nurse and priest, I have walked on a journey into dementia with Christine Bryden, starting soon after her diagnosis. Dementia is still a feared condition and perhaps fear is one of the greatest barriers to living a quality life for those who have dementia. Too often people with dementia are shut off from others in the community and may be even isolated within their own families. It was this factor that really struck me when I began working with Christine. She was the first person that I had really been able to talk with openly about dementia. Previously, I had found that often barriers seemed to exist between the person with dementia and others. Working with Christine challenged me to research the experience of dementia for others as well, with the major questions, such as how can we assist people with dementia to find meaning in their experiences. How can we affirm their personhood?

Dementia as a topic of conversation

For the first time in my professional career as a nurse, I was challenged to meet with Christine as a person first and as someone with dementia, second. Nurses learn how to 'manage' dementia. I contend that dementia is not managed; the best 'management' can leave the person isolated in the middle of this disease. With Christine, I was able to talk freely about dementia; we named it, and we focused on the meaning of it for her. Christine was the centre of our conversations. I was learning how to do this too. I found that it was more important to be a person journeying with her, as a partner, not an expert.

Questions that come with dementia are

'Who am I as I travel into this disease?' Christine asked, 'Who will I be when I die?' (Boden, 1998). 'How long do I have before I lose control?' 'Will I know that I am losing it?' 'What does my life mean now that I have dementia?'

Some people, even care providers in residential aged care facilities, find it hard to speak of dementia to those who have it. I can only say that of those I have worked closely with, the ones who have been able to talk openly of their disease seemed to be better able to experience and live with this disease.

The essence of facilitating well-being and providing effective care when it is required includes the spiritual dimension. This involves walking with the person, to help them reflect on their life meaning and the effects of this disease. It is vitally important to engage with the person with dementia and to individualize their care through good assessment of needs. So, what is spirituality, and how can it be a part of dementia care? This chapter addresses issues of dementia and creative processes to facilitate expressions of spirituality.

What is spirituality?

Over the past couple of decades spirituality has come to be recognized and acknowledged as an important aspect of being human. Prior to the 1990s, spirituality was not often spoken of and little research had been published. Even so, some important early work on spirituality in nursing, including Ruth Stoll's (1979) and Verner Carson's (1989) work set the scene for later research and practice development. A recent book on study on spirituality and ageing has provided evidence of the growing body of research in this field (McFadden et al., 2003). Initially the main interest within spirituality was on palliative care, then it moved to mental health and ageing. Only more recently has the place of spirituality been considered specifically in relation to people with dementia (Killick, 2004; MacKinlay, 2002, 2004, 2006, 2008; MacKinlay & Trevitt, 2006; McFadden et al., 2000).

There are numerous definitions for spirituality; for the purposes of this chapter the definition developed by MacKinlay (2001) will be used: 'That which lies at the core of each person's being, an essential dimension which brings meaning to life' (p. 52). This is further enlarged by acknowledging 'that spirituality is not constituted only be religious practices, but must be understood more broadly, as relationship with God, however God or ultimate meaning is perceived by the person, and in relationship with other people'. This definition is applicable to people who have a religious faith and to those who do not. It is important to see spirituality as a part of each human being, and just as each person chooses how they will develop their physical abilities and potential, the same applies to the psychosocial and spiritual dimensions of the human being. Until recently strategies for addressing matters of the spiritual dimension had been largely underdeveloped. Now it is apparent that activities that involve the spiritual dimension are of value, not only to cognitively competent people but to people with dementia too. In fact, engaging with the spiritual dimension opens an important means of communication and meaning for people with dementia.

In providing appropriate spiritual care, it is important to distinguish between religion and spirituality. Sometimes, people are denied the support of spiritual care because carers incorrectly associate spirituality only with religion, while others may believe that that the spiritual dimension is so personal and individual that it cannot be addressed in providing care. These ideas are being challenged with new evidence from recent research, some of which is described in this chapter.

It is acknowledged here that spiritual care is an important and real component of wholistic care. The spiritual dimension is worked out in a variety of ways by human beings.

A well functioning religion will include all or most of these ways; however, for many people the spiritual dimension will not include any traditional religious practices. A diagram may assist in seeing how the spiritual dimension can be mediated for different people (Figure 11.1).

Spiritual care is now seen to be part of the modalities of care that can be provided by chaplains, nurses, life skills coordinators and activity officers, social care providers and others who work with dementia care. The ways in which spiritual care is delivered will differ according to the professional and vocational roles of the providers, with chaplains and pastoral carers taking a broader role than other health care providers. Strategies for spiritual care can be developed: for example, the sensitive use of humour, and the use of spiritual reminiscence to assist people with dementia to find meaning in their lives and to improve their level of well-being. Concepts and practices of spirituality and spiritual care will be developed in this chapter.

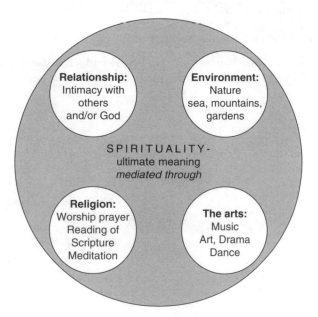

Figure 11.1 Differentiating between religion and spirituality: ways of responding to the spiritual

Source: Adapted from MacKinlay (2006), p. 14.

Spirituality and dementia

Two significant authors in early work on change of culture in dementia care were Kitwood (1997) with his focus on person-centred care and Goldsmith (1996), who asked questions of people with dementia, and their carers, about what they wanted in types of care. Swinton (2001) suggests that asking different questions about dementia can result in a re-framing of attitudes towards dementia. For instance, he writes that if we re-frame the questions of dementia to ask, 'What does it feel like to have dementia, rather than simply, "what is dementia", we begin to see this particular condition in a very different light' (p. 165). Asking the question, 'what does it feel like', is to tap into the spiritual aspect of dementia. This kind of thinking is in line with the work of Kitwood (1997), where the person, not the disease is the focus of care. As Goldsmith wrote (2001a) the new approach to dementia care 'is the insistence on placing the person at the centre, and honouring them and listening to their voice ...' (2001a, p. 125).

A model for spirituality in later life[1]

A model of spirituality may be helpful in creating a framework for understanding the spiritual needs of a person with

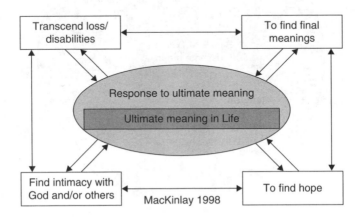

Figure 11.2 A model of spiritual tasks and process of ageing
Source: Adapted from MacKinlay (2001), p. 157.

dementia. A model can assist carers to identify spiritual issues and needs. As dementia mostly occurs in later life, a model of spirituality based on data from in-depth interviews of older people, formed the basis for further research with people with dementia (MacKinlay, 2006; MacKinlay & Trevitt, 2006). The original model developed from work with older people without dementia (MacKinlay, 1998, 2001) was found to also work well for people with dementia.

The model's core consists of meaning as perceived by the older people. The other themes identified in the research were, first, the way that study participants responded to meaning in their lives. This emphasized the importance of what lay at the very centre of their lives. If the participants could see meaning in their lives, then they could respond to that meaning, and life would be worth living. For those who found meaning in their religious faith, their way of worship formed an important component of response to meaning. Others, who found core meaning in human relationships, responded through these relationships. On the other hand, if the person could *not* see meaning in their lives, then life would seem pointless.

The other themes of the model identified from the participants' in-depth interviews were relationship versus isolation, moving from provisional to final life meanings, transcendence of losses and griefs and finding hope (see Figure 11.2). The model is a dynamic one, with feedback to and from the core meaning for the person and interactions with each of the themes.

The model in dementia

Perhaps the greatest challenge to people diagnosed with dementia is their search for meaning leading to the development of effective coping strategies as their memory loss and confusion progresses (Boden, 1998; Goldsmith, 1996). McFadden et al. (2000) noted that older people with dementia seemed to find meaning in their lives and 'repeatedly demonstrated the defiant power of the human spirit' (p. 73).

The importance of ritual for people with dementia in responding to meaning

Humans need ways of responding and connecting with meaning. Rituals and symbols are important vehicles to carry meaning. Even when people with dementia can no longer speak, rituals and symbols may speak powerfully to them. The importance of ritual is to link people with symbols that in turn connect to meaning for the person. Ritual can be played out using symbols, for example a cross, candles, scripture, music or liturgical robes. It is important to be sensitive to what is meaningful for particular people, considering their faith backgrounds, and symbols and rituals that actually mean something to the people involved. Rituals and symbols can be religious or secular.

The search for meaning is one that reaches to the core of human existence, that is the spiritual dimension. It is from our hearts that we find hope and can reach out to friends and family. An important part of this spiritual process is a journey with someone in a trusting relationship, to explore meaning. We can use a process called 'spiritual reminiscence' to explore meaning, either in small groups of people or on a one-to-one basis with a spiritual guide or partner.

Facilitating the search for meaning

Reminiscence work (Bornat, 1994; Gibson, 2004; Haight & Webster, 1995; Webster & Haight, 2002) and spiritual reminiscence use techniques to facilitate the search for meaning. A study, *Finding meaning in the experience of dementia: the place of spiritual reminiscence work*(MacKinlay et al., 2005) examined the process of spiritual reminiscence and how this may be used therapeutically in working with people who have dementia. The project did not examine medical diagnostic processes nor did it address the medical treatment of dementia.

Project objectives were to

- examine how people experience dementia;
- explore how meaning and quality of life can be achieved by and for people who have dementia;

- explore the concept of personhood and respect for persons with dementia;
- develop effective strategies to improve quality of life for those with dementia and
- help families and staff to find meaningful ways to interact with persons who are experiencing communication difficulties in dementia.

The study examined the experience of dementia, the search for meaning and coping strategies used by people with dementia. The project employed phenomenological and grounded theory methods, using small groups, individual interviews and participant observation. In total, 113 people participated in the 27 discussion groups (of 3–6 people). The groups met weekly for 6 weeks or 24 weeks. Demographic data was collected prior to commencement and behaviour ratings were undertaken prior to group commencement and weekly, before and after each group session.

Outcomes of the study

Significant increases in interaction with groups were found on analysis – using Statistical Package for the Social Sciences (SPSS) – of the weekly pre- and post-group behaviour testings, but these changes only became significant from 16th week onwards, indicating the importance of long-term group work with people who have dementia. In analysing the qualitative data from transcripts of weekly sessions using NVivo (a qualitative research computer based analysis program), we often observed participants giving thoughtful answers and showing considerable insight into their situation. The ability of the person to respond was frequently linked to attitudes and communication style of the group facilitator. Research assistant journals recorded instances of participants spontaneously speaking to each other outside the group, making new friends. Within sessions, participants also supported each other through touch and empathetic expression. Although they seemed to lack a sense of time for other activities, some of them would get ready for the group sessions without prompting, and on the right day and time.

People with dementia may need longer to establish relationships, but these friendships seem important to them.
Participants in the longer groups wanted to continue to
keep meeting when the research was over. One group facilitator reported more than a year after the research was completed: 'They eventually knew each other well and formed
friendships, some of which have lasted since (the groups
completed).' Further she said, 'They eagerly came to the
group each week, greeting each other cheerfully and chat-
ting together before the formal questions began. This is not
the norm for many activities with these residents as they are
often not sure what is going on.' Some group members from
the longer groups died and surviving members did grief
work within the group. Members supported each other in
the group.

These groups were an important way of increasing opportunities for interaction and forming new friendships for people with dementia. Group participation seemed not to be
related to the decrease in the Mini Mental State Examination
(MMSE) scores across time. The average MMSE for these
group participants was 18 at the start of the group sessions
and 16 at the conclusion, 24 weeks later. This is important as
some group members continued being in the group until close
to their deaths and, although they continued to deteriorate
in other ways, they still were able to participate in the group.
Obviously, from the data, it can only be assumed that their
ability to continue to engage with others in social skills was
supported by emotional and spiritual well-being, rather than
cognitive abilities. Sessions helped them to find meaning in
their lives and to discuss important issues they were facing,
including loss of loved ones and death.

Relationships In this study, meaning was almost syno-
nymous with relationship. The need for relationship seemed
stronger than with previously studied groups of people who
did not have dementia (MacKinlay, 2001). It is necessary to
move beyond the confusion of words to seek for meaning
in what these people were saying. Family was often not only
important in itself, but gave meaning to the person's whole
existence as well. Sometimes names were forgotten, but there
seemed to be a deeper sense of 'knowing' even though the

person might not be able to state the exact relationship.

Grief Grief was expressed by many; moving into residential aged care was a difficult loss to come to terms with, and it seemed symbolic of many losses: loss of independence and freedom, of control, of belonging and for some, relationship with a spouse who may still be living at home. When my mother was in the final stages of her life, having dementia, when I talked to people about her, they would often ask me 'Does she recognise you?' I found that a confronting question; it was almost as if the expected answer would be 'no'. It seems that this is the wrong question to ask. It assumes a particular understanding of dementia, of a body that no longer has understanding or can be involved in human interactions.

It seems to me that our expectations of the person with dementia are in need of change, as Kitwood (1997) wrote, the onus is on the person without dementia to afford the status of respect and dignity to the one who has dementia. Communication is one of their greatest problems, often in our studies, we found that the search for words was a difficult one. Even if we simply acknowledged that difficulty, the person with dementia would seem to visibly relax, and sometimes, even find the words they wanted. Facial expression is another aspect of the 'knowing'; as we meet and greet people we expect certain facial signs of recognition, a blank face registers as 'she doesn't know me'. In dementia, it is not always possible for the person to adopt the facial expressions that have been customary, thus it is assumed that they do not recognize. We cannot know, therefore it seems more appropriate to act towards the person on the assumption that they may understand more than we might assume.

Image of God For those who held an image of God, the kind of image of God or god held by these people was important to understand in relation to their needs for wholistic care. Not all people held an image of God. There were a variety of images held, some useful in providing hope, others had negative images of God that would not be helpful in providing spiritual support. In providing spiritual care, it is important to be aware of the spiritual needs of the person. One elderly man with dementia, when asked if he had an idea of what God might be like responded, 'The Bible will take me home.' Although he did not directly answer the question, there was no doubt about what his image of God was.

Attending church and private religious practices For some, this was very important, for others it was not important at all. Many of the residents attended church regularly in the facility they lived in. Increasing frailty can make it harder for people to sit through a service of worship. One registered nurse, working in aged care told me that older people were not interested in religion because they didn't go to the church services. The spiritual dimension cannot be assessed solely on the basis of frequency of church attendance. In this study, most of the participants said they prayed. Older people tend to pray differently, some saying that they talk more with God, or they just sit and listen. That is still prayer. In the spiritual reminiscence groups some of the group members spontaneously prayed.

Wisdom and insight This may be surprising to some, but in a number of the responses of these people, there is insight and wisdom, if wisdom is defined more broadly than in the cognitive sense, in a more profound and philosophic way. This broader understanding of wisdom included an increased tolerance to uncertainty, a deepening search for meaning in life, including an awareness of the paradoxical and contradictory nature of reality; it involves transcendence of uncertainty and a move from external to internal regulation (based on Blanchard-Fields & Norris, 1995, p. 108).

Transcendence Many of these people had multiple dis-abilities that made communication even more difficult. Some worried but most said they accepted life as it comes. So, it would seem, there was a sense of transcendence for some of these people.

Hope Hope is critical in finding meaning in life. Hope is an essential ingredient in suicide prevention. Hopelessness is a symptom of depression. The question in the study was, 'What sort of things give you hope in life now?' Most of the responses focused around relationship, seeing their adult children or grandchildren do well, seeing their family. For some hope was tied to their faith, and through prayer. For others, the response to hope was 'nothing very much'.

A guide on spiritual reminiscence A grant from the Wicking Trust made it possible to design, trail and publish a guide for facilitating spiritual reminiscence work for people with dementia, based on the findings of this study (MacKinlay & Trevitt, 2006). The program is being used widely with older people who have dementia.

Humour and dementia One of the observations from the 1998 study and again from the 2002 and 2006 studies of older people, with or without dementia, is the way in which humour is used. All of the participants in the MacKinlay et al. (2002) study had dementia. Instances of humour analysed from the transcripts found that some participants showed evidence of insight. In fact, sometimes during the small group sessions, the cognitively intact facilitator/staff member failed to see or acknowledge instances of humour used by these people who have dementia, and the humour was only apparent when the session transcripts were later transcribed and analysed.

Laughter was often present in the group sessions. The following interchange reflects the sense of fun that some of these people retain and their interaction within the group. The facilitator asked where she could assist them in finding meaning now, resulting in this exchange:

> Dorothy: I find things to interest myself, I read a lot, do exercises, I run up and down my room a hundred times.
> Facilitator: She does, she runs everywhere Bob.
> Bob responds: She's probably got the foundations improved in her home.
> Dorothy: I don't feel my age, until I look in the mirror.
> Bob: You look pretty good too.
> Dorothy: Oh thanks dear and you always look lovely.
> Bob: Thank you. (MacKinlay, 2002, p. 56)

This is part of a transcribed conversation between nursing home residents who have dementia (all names have been changed to protect the individuals). In this exchange, humour could be seen as a means of transcending some of the hard parts of life. The instances were initiated by group members and led to increased interaction in the group.

Is humour just fun, or there is purpose behind it? Is there benefit from humour? In the 1997 edition of Frankl's *Man's Search for Ultimate Meaning*, he wrote of 'two uniquely human capacities of self-transcendence and self-detachment'. (1997, 110) According to Frankl, a technique called paradoxical intention may be used to distance the person from their problem, by 'a unique and specific aspect of self-detachment, namely, the human sense of humour' (p. 110). It is said that in laughing at the problem it distances, and diffuses the topic, 'takes the wind out of the sales' (Frankl 1986, 224–225).

An everyday example using humour by distancing occurs when an older person laughs or jokes at their decreasing mobility, or their forgetfulness. This move comes from within the person; it is not making a joke at someone else's expense. Jokes that emphasize the negative aspects of ageing may be offensive to some older people, yet on the other hand older people may use such stories of failing health against themselves, initiating a humorous anecdote. This has been noticeable in some of the small spiritual reminiscence groups of people who have dementia and are in residential aged care (MacKinlay, 2002). It is interesting that although people in the small groups engaged in conversations around memory loss, and laughed about it, memory loss was identified as part of growing older, rather than dementia. Behind the jokes may lie a fear of memory loss and its possible implications. Thus the use of humour to distance oneself from the feared situation may act to lessen its impact. A sense of humour may facilitate the process of dealing with some of the difficulties encountered in growing older. Humour may be involved in the process of self-transcendence that occurs in some older people; in the model of spiritual task of ageing (MacKinlay, 2006), transcendence is identified as one of the tasks. Further, authentic humour of the spiritually mature person can be acknowledged as conveying a deep sense of trust and hope.

It is important for carers working with older adults to recognize authentic humour in those they work with, and to also learn to use humour appropriately in their own work, taking the lead from those they care for. Inappropriate use of humour appears condescending and demeaning. Spiritual maturity among older people varies greatly, as with people at any age; some older persons have a deeply developed spiritual dimension, while others have focused more on physical and/ or psychosocial aspects of life and come to later life with few spiritual strategies. Spiritual maturity is always a becoming, never an arrival and completion. As I reflected on the use of humour in these studies I wrote,

> It is often said that it takes a long time to develop trust between people. And yet, it must be remembered that in each case that I have discussed here, as researcher, I had only met the informant on one previous occasion. So it would appear that it is possible to develop communication to a deep level of connection and sharing in a relatively short period of time. I am suggesting it is possible to connect deeply, given that you have and use effective listening skills and exercise the ability of being sensitive to the needs of the person you are communicating with. This includes giving the speaker time to express themselves, to reflect on their thoughts and respond knowing that they will be listened to. (MacKinlay, 2002, p. 53)

The trust that can be facilitated in spiritual care is the basis for spiritual growth and an opening to new ways of being when living with dementia. This brings a focus to ask what can I do and be, rather than what I can't do and be. Using a spiritual approach can help the person affirm their identity again. It can go to the core of their being, to strip away the things that are not important, to focus on what is important. The process of spiritual reminiscence always respects and supports the person with dementia. It assists by affirming who they are in this journey, allowing them to share their deepest fears and hopes. It provides a safe place just to 'be'.

To engage with the spiritual dimension in dementia is to provide, not just medical care, but really wholistic care. It will enable the person with dementia to flourish, in spite of their disease or disability. This process of spiritual care is being used more and more widely as part of wholistic care to support people with dementia.

Conclusion

In this chapter, I have focused on two creative approaches to facilitating spiritual well-being and care. The first of these is the use of spiritual reminiscence with people who have dementia. This evidence-based program has positive outcomes for people with dementia and outcomes of the project clearly show improved quality of life for participants. It is emphasized though, that this kind of program should be used in the longer-term care of people with dementia; short groups of around six weeks have not shown significant changes (MacKinlay & Trevitt, 2006). Support groups should be small and have meaningful content for the participants. They are able to develop friendships and increase their social skills within these groups. These kinds of programs assist aged care facilities to provide environments in which people with dementia can be valued and can flourish.

The second creative process described in this chapter, with a spiritual component, is that of humour and its effective use and encouragement with people who have dementia. Further work may help to develop ways that humour can be introduced more effectively when working with older people, in the community and in aged care. Qualitative methods can be used to open up areas of practice that have not been previously studied and where change of practice is needed. Qualitative studies respect the people they study and give people, particularly vulnerable people, a voice.

The issues raised in this chapter are at the heart of what it is to be human. People living with dementia find it hard at times to communicate effectively. All staff in aged care facilities need to be aware of the kinds of difficulties these people experience and be willing to support them in respectful caring environments.

Small group work with people who have dementia can be highly effective in assisting these people to make new friends and to increase their social skills. The setting is important, with an environment of safety and quietness. The ability of small group facilitators to communicate effectively with people with dementia is crucial to the well-being of people with dementia.

There are different kinds of programs being developed for work with people who have dementia. Art and music, singing and pastoral care are all valuable; some study of the effectiveness of such programs has been, and is being done. In some cases, programs are conducted that do not take account of the research already available, and in other cases, lifestyle coordinators/diversional therapists and others who fill these roles have little preparation in developing their knowledge and skills for working with people who have dementia. It is now more than a decade since Tom Kitwood published his work in person-centred care and it seems that the 'new' culture he advocated for is slow in coming. Using the principles of person-centred care makes an incredible difference for the lives and well-being of people with dementia. It is essential that research into the effectiveness of programs and development of new programs, based on research, will be done so that best practice can be achieved.

Education in new strategies for care of people with dementia is the next step. High priority is given to education of staff in ways that will facilitate appropriate communication skills in aged care staff. This should include nurses, leisure skills coordinators, diversional therapists, clergy, social workers, volunteers and all who care for people with dementia. Evidence-based practice must be introduced in care settings. Too often in dementia care, behaviours are still being targeted, rather than affirming the person and working with them. Spiritual reminiscence and the appropriate use of humour interspersed in respectful ways can be affirming and raise morale and a general sense of well-being within a care environment.

Note

1. Further explanation of these models is contained within the book: MacKinlay, E. (2006). *Spiritual Growth & Care in the Fourth Age of Life*. London: Jessica Kingsley Publishers.

References

Blanchard-Fields, F. & Norris, L. (1995). The Development of Wisdom. In M. A. Kimble, S. H. McFadden, J. W. Ellor & J. J. Seeber (eds), *Aging, Spirituality, and Religion: A Handbook*. Minneapolis: Augsburg Fortress Press, 102–118.

Boden, C. (1998). *Who Will I Be when I Die?* Pymble: Harper Collins Religious.

Bornat, J. (ed.) (1994). *Reminiscence Reviewed*. Buckingham: Open University Press.

12 Creative communication at the end of life

John Killick and Kate Allan

Introduction

This is perhaps the most challenging area of creativity to be considered in this book. To aspire to engage people with very profound dementia, as well as physical frailties, in creative activities and to communicate with them in authentic ways may seem very difficult. We are certainly still at the beginning of exploring the possibilities in these circumstances. The literature is small, and initiatives have been tentative, but in our view there are grounds for believing that a great deal is possible and remains to be understood if we have the courage, determination and patience to venture into the unknown.

In what follows we begin by considering some general issues which arise in relation to working with people with profound dementia, then go on to discuss some approaches which have been developed for communicating with persons who present challenges in this respect, for example those with severe autism or individuals in coma. We believe that there is a lot to learn from these 'parallel' situations. The subject of creativity and how we can approach this then follows with some examples.

Getting into a helpful frame of mind

Having the right frame of mind for approaching work with any person with dementia is of course important, but we feel it is necessary to give particular prominence to this subject in relation to working with people who have profound disabilities and are close to the end of their lives.

It seems right to begin this discussion with a point eloquently made in the highly recommended documentary film *There is a Bridge*, which comes from an organization working in creative ways with persons with dementia in Chicago. In the film, Stanley Hauerwas, who is a professor of theological ethics, talks about the subject of presence. He describes the common human tendency, particularly when spending time with someone who is in some way suffering, to focus on *doing*. He says,

> We forget that our most precious gift for one another is presence – just being present.

But what does it mean to be present? A core aspect of this relates to the subject of time; indeed Hauerwas talks about becoming a friend to a person with dementia as 'becoming a friend of time'. Time is a big subject – in every sense! In life generally, and certainly in care settings, the lack of time is often bemoaned. We often seem to be in difficult relationship with the passing of time, feeling that either an unpleasant activity will never end or an enjoyable one passes far too quickly. (For a consideration of the subject of time in relation to supporting people with dementia, see Gilliard & Marshall, 2010.) Is it possible to find a different way of relating to time, and how could this help us when working with persons who are living with advanced dementia?

Perhaps we can learn from those who have direct experience, and who have important things to say about their relationship with time. Cary Smith Henderson (Henderson et al., 1998, p. 41), who was diagnosed with early onset dementia, says,

> Every day is separate.
> You don't know
> What's going to happen
> In any one day.
> It's as if every day
> You have never seen
> Anything before
> Like what you're seeing right now.

If living with dementia increases the saliency of the present moment, then this provides a pointer for how we ourselves should approach this issue. The practice of mindfulness meditation, which comes from Buddhist teachings, has direct relevance here. Jon Kabat-Zinn (2005) describes mindfulness as a discipline which emphasizes the value of 'practising being', 'tuning into the basic experiences of living' and 'being in the moment without trying to change anything'. There is evidence that such experience has a range of benefits in our lives generally, including allowing us to feel less driven by our thoughts, and more connected with our surroundings and being at greater ease with time. Indeed, Kabat-Zinn has described it as a way of 'making time'. If we are to increase our capacity for being with persons with dementia in an authentic and creative way, then this is something which we must develop. Lisa Snyder (2002), who is a social worker with a great deal of experience of working with persons with dementia, said,

> For Bill the past is elusive and the future uncertain. A relationship with him can be demanding – but also deeply inspiring. Like a Zen master he exacts my conscious attention to each present moment and renews my appreciation for the unpredictable and spontaneous dimensions of life.

Exploring the idea of presence further, it seems to us that the quality of openness is essential. If we are to be fully present with another person, and especially one who has so many obstacles to overcome in order to reach out to another, then a heightened quality of openness and availability to that other person is required. If we approach the situation with expectations about what would constitute success, or with a particular endpoint in mind, then we are more likely to pay attention and respond to some things at the expense of others. We may convey a mood of tension if what we want to happen does not, and our sense of the pacing or overall shape of the encounter is likely to be affected. This might mean that we give up too easily or keep going when it is not beneficial to the other person.

Being open demands that we try as fully as possible to appreciate and share what the person is experiencing, and what they are giving during the time we share with them. We need to put any agenda of our own to one side and enter wholeheartedly into the moment. It is difficult to describe such a state, but as well as involving the will to do so, it demands certain skills such as close observation of how the person is in that moment, what they are doing and to what they are giving their attention. Do they seem to be focused on internal experiences, or are they affected by the aspects of the environment such as sounds, temperature, texture and air movement? Entering into the moment with another person also means using one's own experience in an imaginative way whilst being aware of the distinction between what relates to ourselves and what belongs to the other.

The American musician Lois J. McCloskey (1990) provides a description of what this means to her:

> I believe presence is the key element in working with people whose verbal skills are minimal. By presence I mean listening without a particular expectation or a prior agenda. Instead of trying to bring them to my world or orienting them to my 'reality', I allow myself to go where they are and orient myself to their reality. I look deep into their eyes and observe their facial expressions, their body postures, their behaviour. I speak quietly, calmly, and in a non-threatening tone. To do this, I must be focused and free from distractions. We meet in a quiet space without outside noise or interruptions. Because people with dementia are easily over-stimulated and their attention span is difficult to maintain, individual sessions averaging 15 minutes are most effective, though small groups lasting about 30 minutes can also work.

We need to convey the sense that we are accepting of and comfortable with, however the individual is and whatever they are doing. This involves a certain quality of stillness and relaxation, and appropriate responsiveness to what the person offers. This seems to be important for them to take the risk of reaching out, of sharing something of themselves and ultimately having the chance to take the lead in an encounter. Later in the chapter we discuss the practice of mirroring, which is an example of such responsiveness.

It used to be assumed that the words and actions of the person with dementia are generally meaningless, merely the fragmented output of a disordered brain. We have made real progress in terms of challenging such perceptions, and being able to see what an individual says or does as being as meaningful as we would with any other person. Where those with very advanced dementia are concerned, however, there is more often a perception that the individual really has progressed beyond a point where it is possible to see meaning or sense. This is something we have to work to challenge, just as has happened with people with milder disabilities. Being with someone in the context of attempting communication or creative activity is an excellent opportunity to practice such an attitude, to assume that there is a reason, whether or not it is discernible to ourselves, for everything the person does. Only with such a disposition will we be able to value the individual properly and have the chance to connect in a genuine way.

Practical issues

Although it is impossible to generalize, it is often the case that someone who has had dementia for a long time and is nearing the end of their life will appear disengaged from their immediate surroundings, perhaps with their eyes closed even when awake, and with their body turned in on itself in an almost foetal position. They may seem unaware of what is happening around them, appear to ignore remarks addressed to them and behave passively when someone touches them, moves them or undertakes care tasks. There may also be sudden sounds or movements from the person which do not seem related to anything happening around them.

For someone who is relatively immobile, activities are more likely to have to be something which can be brought to them, rather than relying on being in a space dedicated to creative work. This may constrain what is attempted, but many activities can be simplified and made portable, for example on a tray or easily manoeuvrable table. And keeping things simpler and limiting what is presented may actually be more suitable for someone with very complex disabilities. Attention to physical comfort is essential, and in such situations it is likely that shorter sessions will be more successful than longer ones.

The health and safety implications of activities may have to be re-evaluated for an individual in this situation. In particular it is important to remember that the person may be more likely to attempt to put objects or materials in their mouth.

In general, the kinds of actions initiated or responses made by such an individual are likely to be more subtle than those with less profound disabilities. A facial expression may be extremely fleeting and only partial, such as a flicker of the eyebrows or a twitch of the mouth. Another part of the body may be moved, or a sound uttered which is difficult to distinguish from a sigh or a cough. It may be difficult to know whether things the person does are voluntary or involuntary. In these circumstances it is necessary to adopt a lower threshold of sensitivity to possible responses, and to cultivate an awareness of the effects of the environment on the person. Looking for subtle signals of what is interesting to the person, for example, through eye pointing, can be an important way of making a connection.

It may also be that there is a time delay between a stimulus and a response, and so we need to have a wider 'frame' in which to try to make sense of what is going on. The practice of focusing on the moment and being open and available to the person is especially pertinent to these sorts of situations, and the kind of approaches to interaction which are described later in this chapter are particularly suitable.

On account of the minimal nature of the person's actions and responses, in many situations, greater proximity to the person than that which usually feels normal will be required. At first this may feel uncomfortable both from one's own point of view and also because it is not clear whether the other person welcomes such closeness, and vigilance for expressions of discomfort is important. However, it is also important to allow time for the person to adjust to what is probably a new situation for them, and not react too quickly by withdrawing or assuming that the situation is not acceptable. Making these judgements is not easy, and some risk-taking is necessary.

Most older people have sensory disabilities which affect their ability and opportunities for communication. A study in which Kate was involved explored the implications of deafness combined with dementia, both acquired hearing loss and profound or cultural deafness (Allan, 2006), but in general the effects of sensory loss in combination with dementia remains a neglected area. For persons with especially profound dementia, we must be mindful that sensory needs will have a greater impact on the person's communication resources and we need to find ways to support them as much as possible.

Related to the subject of sensory loss is sensory deprivation. Persons with very advanced dementia, and probably also more complex physical care needs, are more likely to live in institutions than normal domestic environments. This raises a variety of issues which have a bearing on creative activity and experience. Although there have been great advances in understanding about the effects of the physical environment on people with dementia, sadly most institutional settings are still dominated by the needs of staff to care for the physical needs of the person. It is usual to find people at a very advanced stage of dementia spending most of their time in bed or in chairs in rooms either with bare walls nearby or positioned so far from walls that pictures and the like are effectively unavailable. Their posture may mean that their usual view is of floor coverings, chair legs and the feet of people passing by, or of the ceiling. Other than clothes or bedclothes, it is likely that there will be nothing interesting within reach to touch. It is not uncommon for a television to be turned on, but again positioned quite far from the individual and without any special regard for their preferences. Any music is more likely to reflect the tastes of staff than individuals with dementia. Extraneous noise may be an issue, coming either from other persons with dementia or from staff interacting with one another, or (in old buildings) sounds of banging doors, trolleys and so on resounding off hard surfaces.

Occupational therapist Claire Craig has written about how we can understand and transform environments with reference to the subject of creativity (Craig, 2002), and she draws attention to the all-important theme of relationship:

> During the course of my work with people with dementia I came to learn that the environment in which a person lives is about so much more than a physical space. It is about a relationship – the relationship a person has with their surroundings. In this space the belongings people have aren't just about decoration, they are often expressions of style, of the story behind the object, of meanings and memories and a representation of the freedom to exercise choice and to be.

Particular challenges

To encounter someone who appears remote, detached or even unreachable, and attempting to engage with them, is an especially demanding activity which requires a lot of resources. Here we are faced with the extremes of human experience and this is inevitably unsettling. We are confronted with the reality that this is how life is for many people, known and unknown, and how it may be at the end for our loved ones and ourselves. In such a context it is likely that strong feelings will arise, including perhaps sadness, guilt, anger, helplessness and fear. Acknowledging these feelings and accepting them as natural is important, whilst at the same time not becoming so overwhelmed by them that it is impossible to focus on the other person. Experience is a factor in being able to negotiate this, and for anyone attempting such work it is essential that there are regular opportunities for reflection on one's experience. This should include being able to talk with another person who understands the importance of what is being done and the need for support in making sense of it.

However, it is inevitable, at least at times, that we will struggle with doubts about what we are doing: whether it is meaningful, whether it is welcomed by the other person and whether it is a good use of limited resources. As well as our own internal struggles with such concerns, it is likely, especially in institutional settings, that others will have views on these issues. They may comment sceptically on what is being done, even going so far as to dismiss efforts, pouring scorn on the whole idea of trying to connect with someone so disabled and implying that time is being wasted that could be used in more worthwhile activities. Even if such things are not said out loud, when we feel vulnerable about what we are doing, it is easy to assume that others are thinking the worst. It hardly needs pointing out that all this is anathema to the enterprise of trying to enter into the world of the person with advanced dementia and communicate creatively with them.

There is no easy answer to such problems, and often others' attitudes will only change when they see results, and even then only if they are open to having their minds changed. But because this is a shadowy and ill-defined area of work, and one where what seems like clear-cut responses can be downplayed by others, it is especially important that anyone working in this way is clear about their own beliefs, motivations and hopes. Having a clear personal rationale underpinning one's efforts, and linking this with other personal values seems vital. Using 'reference points' such as rehearsing examples of successful work (our own or others') and recalling the encouragement of others are useful strategies. Confidence and resilience to discouragement will grow with experience if this is usefully reflected on and supported by others. We conclude this section with a favourite quotation from hospital chaplain Debbie Everett (1996):

> We must not fear the unknown, or the insufficiency or powerlessness we feel when we are with someone with dementia. Yes, we can experience it, but we must not allow the fear to keep us away. The powerlessness that may occur when caring for a person with dementia has a lot to do with the caregiver's inability to value other means of communication than just words. This fear multiplies the feeling of meaninglessness about ministering to these people. When we see only meaninglessness, commitment is often lost. Surrender to the mystery of the future means admitting the possibility of suffering. Real care for those affected by dementia only takes place when the walls of fear have been removed.

Frameworks for interacting with persons with advanced dementia

Although not concerned specifically with creative activities, some approaches have been developed for working with people who have profound disabilities, and it is appropriate to mention them here as they have the potential to provide a more general framework for interaction, and therefore for undertaking creative activities.

Phoebe Caldwell works in the UK with people with severe learning disabilities, including individuals with autistic spectrum disorders, and uses an approach called 'Intensive Interaction' (Caldwell, 2008). This approach involves focusing on what the person is doing in the present moment, by 'mirroring' their sounds and movements as a way of establishing a relationship and communicating with them. By using this approach she has had much success in connecting meaning-fully with individuals who have been 'written off' as unreach-able by others. She has published books and DVDs which describe and illustrate the approach, and further investigation of her approach will pay dividends to those seeking to extend their skills.

Inspired by this and other work, Maggie Ellis in the UK has recently undertaken a PhD study into the use of such an approach with persons with advanced dementia, and writes about the importance of imitation in interactions with a woman who had severe dementia and struggled with mean-ingful conversation (Ellis & Astell, 2008).

Related to these approaches is something we ourselves have experience of using with persons who are nearing the end of life and have had dementia for a long period. This is called 'coma work' (Mindell, 1999) and was developed as a way of communicating with individuals who are in coma, typically after sudden brain injury. It has elements in common with Intensive Interaction in that close observation of the person's actions and physical state and mirroring of actions and sounds are central. But what is distinctive about this way of working is specific attention to the way the person is breathing, and efforts to match this style of breathing oneself. This sounds simple but is in fact very demanding, and can be challeng-ing especially if the person is breathing very quickly or slowly. When other forms of communication are used, such as sing-ing or humming or the use of touch, these are linked with the person's breathing. So, in the case of touch, gentle pressure may be applied on the person's hand or arm in time with their way of breathing. If a communication partner is speaking or singing to the person, they would again adopt the rhythm of the person's breathing in pacing this. This attention to basic physiological rhythms has the potential to open up an even more profound way of sharing the person's experience and connecting with them.

The 'coma work' approach was not designed with people with dementia in mind, but Tom Richards and Stan Tomandl (2006), who were trained by the Mindells, describe using a variant called 'Process Work' with Stan's father, Stanley, who had had dementia for many years. Over the four years or so before his death, Tom and Stan visited him regularly in the nursing home where he lived, and used various communicative strategies. Despite the severity of his disabilities, Stanley responded by squeezing their hands and at times using clearly meaningful speech, eye contact, joining in with singing and expressive gestures. Their book, *An Alzheimer's Surprise Party*, is so called because of the final celebration of Stanley's life, in which he took a very active part, only 24 hours before he died.

Our own experience of using such an approach during a project in Australia was extremely interesting. A fuller account of this can be found in Killick and Allan (2005, 2006a, 2006b). We, and those who had known the participants over many years, were particularly struck by the instances of clearly meaningful communication, often taking a considerable time to achieve and lasting only a short time, but nevertheless having a highly distinctive and significant character. The work also raised various ethical issues. John has reflected on the very demanding nature of this activity for himself as the active communication partner, how much energy it took to connect and how difficult it was to disconnect having achieved this, especially if the other person seemed still to have a need to remain in communication despite being physically unable to sustain it. These reflections remind us that we are vulnerable too, and that there are dangers in attempting intimate communication work without proper supervision and support (Killick, 1999).

Creative activities

If all this seems extremely complex and demanding, that is because it is! And this is before we even attempt any kind of creative activity! But what kind of creative activities are possible with someone in this situation? Is it realistic at all? Certainly we have to adopt a much wider definition of what constitutes creativity and what counts as communication than is normally in use. We will often be referring to small acts: a mark made on paper or a sound uttered, for instance, rather than a finished art object or complete statement. It is largely a frontier of gestures and approximations, full of uncertainties and bafflements. To enter the realm of creative communication in advanced dementia we must leave dogmatism outside and embrace mystery largely as the norm. A practical consequence of this is that the kind of activities we attempt will need to adopt the same kind of openness as described above. Rather than having a particular plan in mind, we will need to be ready to respond to the person in the moment we find them, and be willing to go with whatever seems right for them at that time. In what follows we describe some examples of work which can illuminate the possibilities.

Using objects

A project which concentrated on objects was carried out by Angela Byers (1995), an art therapist in the United States of America. Over a considerable period of time, she had noticed that many persons with dementia became very absorbed with items which they found around them and some began collecting them. Seeing this as a creative process, she set out to observe it in detail. She collected a variety of materials, including different kinds of paper, samples of cloth, stones, small plastic containers some with lids, string, sticky tape, gumstrip paper, a pencil and balsa wood. These were laid out in a private room for the therapist and the person with dementia to visit together. Where a person was not mobile a selection of objects was taken to them on a tray. She worked with two women and two men and had sessions of up to 45 minutes with each.

Case study

Here is a part of a description of one of the interactions with Mrs D who was 90 years old:
    She folded and smoothed paper saying 'Crease it, crease it'. She examined objects, looking under lids, stirring in a pot, sometimes showing them to me. Sometimes...she hid things, under paper or cloth. Once, finding herself unable to untangle a piece of ribbon, she hid it, thus putting the problem out of sight and out of mind, hiding from others what she probably felt was a lack of skill. She wrapped up some scissors to make a parcel which she then tucked under her cardigan and took back with her to the ward. I got it back from her, in order to retrieve the scissors, only at a moment when she had forgotten about its importance. The next week I showed it to her, without the scissors, and she wrapped it again making it tighter and neater

---

> and then sat clutching it and dozing off. It was evident that these par-
> cels were important to her; I thought of them as transitional objects
> which retained part of the session in a way in which her memory
> could not.

A wide range of creative processes were engaged in by all four individuals:

Objects were covered, hidden, wrapped, picked up, examined, put in the mouth and moved round the lips; containers were explored on the inside and had things put inside them; paper and cloth were smoothed and folded; rooms were explored, furniture was moved, doors were pulled at and walls were pushed.

The various analyses which Byers makes of these acts are fascinating, but heavily dependent on psychoanalytic theory. However, some clear principles emerge. First, once the materials have been chosen and supplied, the facilitator allows the individual to make choices; this experience of being 'in charge' is one rarely offered to persons with dementia, particularly when normal communication is so difficult. Second, some of the activities may relate to previous occupation, but others could be better understood as symbolic play. Third, there is little sense of the development of a process towards a goal, but there is a strong element of appreciation of the moment in what is experienced. The presence of the facilitator is seen as a constantly reassuring presence, thus giving permission to the individual to experiment. At the same time Byers stresses how important it is for the facilitator to keep a sense of his/her own self in addition to entering into the world of the person with whom they are working.

Music

It is well known that music is one of the most powerful means of communicating with persons with dementia, whatever the severity of the condition. We have many accounts from carers, professional staff and musicians which attest to the fact that people with even profound difficulties respond to music, often surprising others when they tap rhythms, mouth words or even sing out. It is a view that receives powerful endorsement from the neurologist Oliver Sacks in his book *Musicophilia* (2007). He claims that music has the power to

address the emotions, cognitive powers, thoughts, and memories, the surviving 'self' of the patient, to stimulate these and bring them to the fore. It aims to enrich and enlarge existence, to give freedom, stability, organization, and focus.

We know from research carried out in Scandinavia that people with even the most severe disabilities who are bedbound and very limited in their ability to express themselves (Norberg et al., 1986) respond more fully to music compared with other forms of stimulation, such as presenting objects or touching their body. This provides support for the idea that music is a significant tool in communicating with those with dementia near the end of their lives.

Helen Finch (2000) has described how her mother, who had been a keen musician before the onset of dementia, was hospitalized and lost the power of speech. She tapped her daughter's hand in a rhythm that was recognized as 'The Skye Boat Song'. Helen interpreted this as the expression of a wish to be elsewhere. Over the next year Helen's mother sang (but wordlessly) over 20 well-known songs, including, after she had suffered another medical setback, 'The Funeral March'. On the third occasion she sang this she stopped in the middle, which Helen felt was a recognition on her mother's part that the message had already been understood and therefore needed no repetition.

An example of an especially instructive, creative and very special interaction comes from the DVD *There Is a bridge* (TMK Productions & Memory Bridge, 2007). It features a woman with advanced dementia called Gladys Wilson and the well-known contributor to the field of communication with persons with dementia, Naomi Feil. In this sequence, we see Gladys Wilson sitting in a chair with her eyes almost closed, slowly tapping her hand on the arm of the chair and moving her legs back and forward slightly. She appears disengaged from her surroundings, existing in her own separate world. On encountering such a person, many would doubt whether anything meaningful was going on in Gladys's mind and whether it was worthwhile to attempt to connect with her. Naomi believes such a person 'will withdraw inward more and more', and 'their desperate need for connection is all now inside'.

Naomi approaches Gladys from the front and greets her with 'Hello, Mrs Wilson'. She is face to face with her, and there is only about 18 inches between them. Gladys reaches up and touches her shoulder. Naomi interprets this as a request for her to sit and confirms this by saying 'Do you want me to sit?' She crouches down to Gladys's level and continues the encounter. There is no space here to describe it blow by blow, but as the interaction unfolds it involves Gladys holding Naomi's hand and moving it in a rhythmic repetitive way. Naomi provides a simplified commentary on what is happening, mentioning that Gladys has a tear on her cheek and touching it gently. She comments that Gladys seems to have pain in her face when she flinches and that her face looks sad. She asks Gladys, 'Is it scary? Are you afraid?', and goes on to touch Gladys's cheekbones, stroking them slowly on both sides. Naomi believes that this kind of touch represents the comfort of being touched by one's mother as an infant and that the body holds such memories thus providing a way of connecting with a person at an elemental level.

Once the encounter is definitely underway, Naomi asks Gladys 'Can you let me in a little?' and at this point, the movement of Gladys's hand on the arm of the chair becomes much more emphatic and rapid. Knowing that Christian songs hold great meaning for her, Naomi begins to sing 'Jesus loves me'. Following on from the very pronounced movement of Gladys's arm, there is an immediate slowing of the rhythm of this to match the speed at which Naomi is singing, very much in the spirit of accompaniment. As the singing goes on, a fascinating dynamic develops whereby Gladys controls the pace and strength of Naomi's singing by the movement of her tapping. Naomi describes a moment here in this way: 'pretty soon we became one person'. Interestingly, Naomi comments that she has been matching her breathing to Gladys's. There is a point where Gladys pulls Naomi towards her and they are forehead to forehead. The sequence concludes with more singing from Naomi, and the climax – which has to be seen to be appreciated – is truly uplifting and inspiring.

In reflecting on this encounter, Naomi warns us that it does not always happen in this way, that there is not always such a profound connection made. But she encourages us:

> But if you keep trying, and you keep centring yourself, and really look at that person, and really mirror their movements, maybe not this time, but the next time you come you'll have a communication. (TMK Productions & Memory Bridge, 2007)

A good sunset

We end with an example of creativity from someone with advanced dementia which involves words, something that becomes increasingly elusive for people in this situation. The following poem which John heard sung during a visit to a facility reminds us of perhaps the biggest challenge we all face – how we can help persons with advanced dementia to have a good death. The lady was sitting in a corner of a nursing home and singing in a controlled but delicate manner. Curious to hear more, John approached her and began close listening. He asked her permission to write down the words she was singing, and she nodded assent. Neither the words nor the melody were familiar, and he concluded that the song was improvised. It seemed to be a spontaneous outpouring of feeling, and an attempt to come to terms creatively with her situation:

> I don't know what to do
> I want to go home
> I can sit here but
> I don't seem happy any more
> I don't know what to do
> I want to but
> I can't any more
> I want to lay
> I don't know when it'll be
> I want it so let me have it
> Don't make it so hard for me
> O World, I don't know what to do
> I want to see my sunset
> I want it as it was promised
> I'm waiting for the hour
> I want to see my sunset good

Conclusion

Whilst this chapter has highlighted some of the challenges in working creatively with persons with advanced dementia, we hope that it has also illustrated that once an adjustment is made, an attuning to what we often overlook in our preoccupation with outcomes, that there is real meaning and connection to be found, and that this can point the way to more creative ways of living for us all.

References

Allan, K. (2006). Deafness and dementia: consulting on the issues. *Journal of Dementia Care*, 14(3), 35–37.

Byers, A. (1995). Beyond marks: on working with elderly people with severe memory loss. *Inscape*, 1(13–18), 15–17.

Caldwell, P. (2008). *Using Intensive Interaction and Sensory Integration: A Handbook for Those Who Support People with Severe Autistic Spectrum Disorder.* London: Jessica Kingsley.

Craig, C. (2002). *Creative Environments: A Practical Approach to Arts Activities.* Stirling: DSDC.

Ellis, M. P. & Astell, A. J. (2008). A Case Study of Adaptive Interaction: A New Approach to Communicating with People with Advanced Dementia. In S. Zeedyk (ed.), *Techniques for Promoting Social Engagement in Individuals with Communicative Impairments.* London: Jessica Kingsley.

Everett, D. (1996). *Forget Me Not: The Spiritual Care of People with Alzheimer's.* Edmonton: Inkwell Press (p. 42)

Finch, H. (2000). Musical keys to communication. *Pathways*, 2(1), 1.

Gilliard, J. & Marshall, M. (2009). *Time for Dementia.* London: Hawker Publications.

Main, J. H., Andrews, N. & Henderson, R. D. (1998). *Partial View: An Alzheimer's Journal.* Dallas, TX: Southern Methodist University Press (p. 41)

Kabat-Zinn, J. (2005). *Full Catastrophe Living: Using the Wisdom of Your Body and Mind to Face Stress, Pain and Illness.* New York: Bantam Dell (p. 20)

Killick, J. (1999). Pathways through pain – a cautionary tale. *Journal of Dementia Care*, 7(1), 22–24.

Killick, J. & Allan, K. (2005). The good sunset project: quality of life in advanced dementia. *Journal of Dementia Care*, 13(6), 22–23.
Killick, J. & Allan, K. (2006a). The good sunset project: making contact with those close to death. *Journal of Dementia Care*, 14(1), 22–24.
Killick, J. & Allan, K. (2006b). The good sunset project: inside the interactions. *Journal of Dementia Care*, 14(2), 27–29.
McCloskey, L. J. (1990). The silent heart sings. *Generations: Counselling and Therapy*, Winter, 63–65.
Mindell, A. (1999). *Coma, A Healing Journey: A Guide for Family, Friends and Helpers*. Portland, OR: Lao Tse Press.
Norberg, A., Melin, E. & Asplund, A. (1986). Reactions to music, touch and object presentation in the final stage of dementia. An exploratory study. *International Journal of Nursing Studies*, 23(4), 315–323.
Richards, T. & Tomandl, S. (2006). *An Alzheimer's Surprise Party: New Sentient Communication Skills and Insights for Understanding and Relating to People with Dementia*. Glenview, IL: Lulu Publishing Inc (available from www.lulu.com) (accessed on 16 January 2011).
Sacks, O. (2007). *Musicophilia: Tales of Music and the Brain*. New York: Knopf (p. 336–337)
Snyder, L. (2002). *Speaking Our Minds: Personal Reflections from Individuals with Alzheimer's*. New York: W. H. Freeman (p.56)
TMK Productions & Memory Bridge (2007). *There is a bridge* (DVD).

Conclusion

Hilary Lee

This book has discussed how person-centred creative approaches and arts provide a significant role in sustaining personhood in dementia care. We have heard from creative pioneers about diverse approaches that bring out the human potential and dormant abilities, and provide new ways for people with dementia to communicate and express their emotions and their inner selves.

A common element in each creative approach described is the insistence that the person is the focus, not the diagnosis, and that the individual in his or her uniqueness is honoured with deep respect. Creativity creates a bridge between the inner and outer world where a new outlet is provided for expression of thoughts and feelings that have been locked away. In a safe psychological space these emotions are freed and expressed in new ways. This book has shown that both creative approaches and the arts have a remarkable power to restore a broken spirit, or damaged self- esteem, to build confidence, gain resolution to life experiences and to realize oneself as an important and valued person. As Kirstin Robertson-Gillam tells us with her story about Bert, the arts (in this case music) can even help in passing from this world to the next.

How do we bring these creative approaches to the attention of people developing dementia policies to direct funds into the regular provision of creative opportunities? One way is to create a groundswell of support for this new way of thinking about dementia care through books such as this to give students and people working in health care some inspiration and new perspectives. Another way is through organizations such as the Society for the Arts in Dementia Care who promote networking and collaboration between creative artists, therapists, health professionals, researchers, seniors with dementia and the community. This organization has played an active role in raising awareness of the value of creative expression for older people with dementia to the community and to health care providers through art exhibitions, workshops and international conferences since 2005. Originally founded by Dr Dalia Gottlieb-Tanaka in Vancouver, British Columbia, the Society was inspired by and based on her PhD, *Dementia, Creativity and the Therapeutic Environment*. The Society was then brought to Australia in 2006 by this author. In addition to the associations for the different arts therapies, new arts groups are emerging in different countries to breathe life, joy and creativity into the worlds of older people with dementia. These include Dementia Positive (UK), ElderClowns (UK), LaughterBoss (Australia) The National Center for Creative Ageing (New York) and The Creativity Discovery Corps at the Centre for Aging, Health and Happiness (Washington).

Currently the creative arts are not implemented in all aged care facilities or community centres. They are often embraced on a project by project basis, depending on available funding. This means that a highly successful project may have to cease due to lack of funds to continue. Groups such as The Society for the Arts in Dementia Care (www.cecd-society.org) operate internationally, providing a united voice for people with dementia to have a right to consistent access to the arts to enrich their lives.

This book has given many examples of the deep meaning that creativity brings to people's lives. In residential care, creative programmes such as those described in this book can add a whole extra dimension to the provision of activities. In particular they add the spiritual dimension where meaning and purpose in life can be explored and manifested.

The creative arts also contribute to enriching relationships by enabling those around the person to understand their world, thoughts, and experiences in new ways. These insights enable practitioners and family carers to be appreciative of the wisdom people with dementia offer us from their life experience and learnings.

This book has given us a glimpse of the unlimited possibilities creativity offers to people with dementia. Looking to the future, we are moving into the unknown. How can we create the future we would like to see? Can we as therapists, health professionals and carers of people with dementia, build a future where people with dementia can access skilled facilitators? How can we support these facilitators to provide the safe psychological environment and to deeply engage with the person to facilitate their freedom and desire to be creative? There is a need to continue researching these new approaches as well as promote the research that has already been undertaken to awaken awareness of the value of the arts to academics, policy makers and the community.

Creativity expands our mind and our options, linking one human spirit to another. For people with dementia creative approaches open up new ways of expression and connection. The creative process holds the power for all of us to achieve our dreams through the door to our imagination. The words of an 80-year-old person with dementia illustrate this point, in a poem by John Killick:

Paragliding at eighty

There were three of us
in the boat, and I was the first
to do it. It was the flying,
it was the feeling free.
And when I flowed like that
I was astonished. And then
I flew again: ONE. TWO, THREE!
When are we going to do it again?
(Killick, 2008, p. 42)

Reference

Killick, J. (2008). *Dementia Diary*. London: Hawker.

Index